P9-BZF-483

Taking Control

Living with the Mitral Valve Prolapse Syndrome

Kristine A. Bludau Scordo, PhD, RN
Assistant Professor, Wright State University
Clinical Director, The Mitral Valve Prolapse Program of Cincinnati

SECOND EDITION
Revised and Updated

Taking Control: Living with the Mitral Valve Prolapse Syndrome.

Copyright ©1996 by K.A. Scordo.

All rights reserved. Printed in the United States of America. No part of this publication may be used or reproduced in any manner whatsoever without written permission except for brief quotations embodied in critical articles and reviews. For information, write The MVP Program of Cincinnati, P.O. Box 626, Loveland, OH 45140.

Publishing History
First Edition: Copyright © 1991 Camden House, Inc.
Graphic Images Copyright © New Vision Technologies Inc.

Library of Congress Cataloging-in-Publication Data

Scordo, Kristine A. Bludau, 1947–
Taking Control: Living with the Mitral Valve Prolapse Syndrome /
Kristine A. Bludau Scordo
      p. cm.
      Includes bibliographical references and index.
      ISBN 0-9650689-0-0 (acid-free)
      1. Mitral valve—Displacement—Popular works.   I. Title

Published by Kardinal Publishing
Designed and produced by GYAT

Printed in the United States of America
ISBN 0-9650689-0-0

Dedication

To those with mitral valve prolapse.

May it do you much good.
—Kaplan, 1964

Contents

Contributors
and Consultants

Kristine A. Bludau Scordo PhD, RN

Assistant Professor Wright State University-Miami Valley, College of Nursing and Health; Clinical Director, The MVP Program of Cincinnati, The Health Promotion and Rehabilitation Center,Cincinnati, Ohio; Clinical Nurse Specialist, Clinical Consultant,The Cardiology Center of Cincinnati,Cincinnati, Ohio

LeOna Kriesel Cox, BS Education

Educator & Author; Former High School Business Teacher; Former Teacher, Economics Department, Allegheny College, Meadville, Pennsylvania; Author of Educational Texts and Filmstrip Scripts

Fuheid S. Daoud, MD

Cardiologist; Medical Director, The Cardiology Center of Cincinnati, The Mitral Valve Prolapse Program of Cincinnati, The Health Promotion and Rehabilitation Center, Cincinnati, Ohio

Linda Harte Hoffsis, MA

Exercise Physiologist; Coordinator of the Cardiac Rehabilitation Program, Health Promotion and Rehabilitation Center, Cincinnati, Ohio; Staff Exercise Physiologist, MVP Program of Cincinnati; Dietetic Student, University of Cincinnati

Linda Hussey, MSN, RN, CS, LPCC

Clinical Nurse Specialist; Psychiatric Nursing; Private Practice, Cincinnati, Ohio

Preface

Since the initial publication of *Taking Control* in 1991, thousands of letters poured in from all over the world. Each week I continue to receive several similar to these:

"More than any physician with whom I consulted, your book gave me a wealth of information and insight into my problem. If only I had this book in 1984 when I was initially diagnosed, how different my life might have been."

"I feel absolutely overwhelmed trying to express my gratitude to you for this most informative book. You've done a great service for MVPers and their families. I can't thank you enough."

"I couldn't put this book down. In Chapter 2, I identified with many of the people who shared their experiences. You'll never know how much this book helped me."

"I can't begin to tell you what a blessing this book is. I've told co-workers, friends, and physicians to read it so they, too, can learn more about MVPS."

Many readers express relief upon learning they're not alone. Fears, feelings, and sometimes frightening experiences are the rule not the exceptions.

Furthermore, your suggestions, as well as data collected from your responses to a questionnaire in the first edition, helped me to revise this updated edition of *Taking Control*. To all of you, I say, "Thank you. Your input enabled *me* to better understand what is genuinely helpful to *you*. For this I am extremely grateful."

To repeat a sentence from the first edition, "This type of book is not possible without the assistance of several individuals." I have the good fortune to work with Mrs. LeOna Kriesel Cox, who is not only an excellent teacher, but also a very gracious woman. I thank her for her wise and tireless editorial assistance, her involvement and sense of pride in the book, and most of all, the energy and enthusiasm with which she approaches her work.

I acknowledge Fuheid S. Daoud, MD for his excellent critique of Chapter 1, and also for his critique of many *Network* newsletters. These newsletters provided helpful information given in Chapter 8.

I am grateful to Linda Harte Hoffsis, MA, staff exercise physiologist at The MVP Program of Cincinnati, and to Linda Hussey, RN, MSN, LPCC, clinical nurse specialist in Cincinnati for reviews of their original contributions, Chapters 4 and 5.

Special acknowledgement goes to James Hardin, PhD and his wife, Anne, from Camden House Publishing. I thank them for their continued belief in this subject.

I am grateful for the assistance of my sisters, Stephanie and Elissa. I thank Stephanie J. Bludau Tor for her encouragement, guidance, and, with her husband, Terrance Tor, for assistance in preparation of the book. I thank Elissa K. Bludau Engelhardt for her review of the manuscript. To my best investment, Lisa, I thank her for the endless hours she spent compiling data from the first-edition questionnaires. I cherish her love and support. And, I wish to acknowledge the support and love from Bob, my significant other.

— *Kristine Scordo*

Foreward
to the First Edition

Taking Control: Living with the MVPS is intended to help individuals to cope with the myriad of symptoms associated with MVPS. Those of us in the medical field frequently diagnose people with this syndrome recognize the enormous and time-consuming difficulty in dealing with the disproportionate perception of these individuals of the serious nature of their symptoms. They are understandably frightened by chest pain, alarmed by palpitations, dizziness, lightheadedness and frustrated by unexplained fatigue, moodiness, and anxiety attacks.

I am afraid that as physicians we have failed to adequately handle the needs of the large number of people with this syndrome, mainly because of the inordinate amount of time it takes to do so. Explaining the common denominator in this syndrome, namely the anatomic variant structure of the valve and support structures, is an easy task. Explaining the varied and multiple associated symptoms, however, is a difficult one. Reassuring these individuals that the chest pain is not necessarily a prelude to a fatal heart attack, that the palpitations are not a signal of a life-threatening arrhythmia, and that the fatigue, tiredness, and headache are not symptoms of underlying serious illness requires a separate and distinct discussion.

Kris Scordo has succeeded in meeting this challenge in *Taking Control*. In addition to her own enormous contribution based on experience gained over several years of clinical experience and research for her doctoral dissertation, she was able to enlist the talent and expertise of others who for years also patiently and tirelessly worked with individuals with this syndrome. She and her colleagues have addressed various aspects of this syndrome, making this book the most comprehensive to date. Individuals with this syndrome should, after reading this book, be able to put the syndrome in proper perspective. I look forward to making it available to every person diagnosed with this syndrome.

Fuheid S. Daoud, MD
Director of Cardiology
Bethesda Hospitals
Cincinnati, Ohio

Acknowledgments to the First Edition

A book of this nature would not have been possible without the assistance of several individuals. I have been very fortunate to work with Fuheid Daoud, MD who is not only an excellent cardiologist and outstanding clinician, but also a gentleman. It was he who first stimulated my interest in MVPS. The MVP Program would not have been possible without his support. I thank him for his excellent suggestions and critique of this book.

I thank Linda Harte Hoffsis, MA, staff exercise physiologist at The MVP Program of Cincinnati, and Linda Hussey, RN, MSN, LPCC, clinical nurse specialist in Cincinnati for contributing Chapters, 4, 5, and 6 to this book.

Appreciation is extended to Lauren Niemes, RD for her review of Chapter 5; James Hawkins, MD for his review of Chapter 6; and to Charles Young, PharmD for his review of Chapter 7. Their comments and suggestions were very helpful.

Linda Hoffsis, Mike Frank, and Nancy Homan, staff at the Health Promotion and Rehabilitation Center, provided invaluable assistance in their thoughtful critique and ideas for the various chapters. I am indebted to Beth White MS, medical librarian, for her thorough review of the literature and for obtaining the many articles and books needed to compile this work. Special acknowledgement goes to Don Wilson, "the ancient artist," who provided the art work.

Special thanks go to the many people with MVPS who reviewed and critiqued the book. Finally, my sincere gratitude goes to the individuals who served as participants in the MVP research study and gave so generously of their time. I learned much from them.

Special recognition goes to my parents who taught me the value of an education and that where there is a will, there is a way. To my daughter, Lisa, who lived this experience as much as I, go my thanks for her love, patience, understanding, and encouragement.

Kristine A. Bludau Scordo, PhD, RN
Clinical Nurse Specialist
The Cardiology Center of Cincinnati;
Clinical Director
The MVP Program of Cincinnati, Ohio

Introduction
to the First Edition

After working several years in a critical-care setting, I joined a group of cardiologists as a clinical nurse specialist. This was over ten years ago. I remember several individuals diagnosed with mitral valve prolapse — MVP — and listening to their stories. Not being well versed on the subject, I began to research the literature to learn all I could about MVP. In particular, I was interested in understanding what causes symptoms in people with MVP. For instance, I noticed that during graded exercise treadmill testing, people with MVP had an inappropriate increase in their heart rate. It wasn't unusual to the see heart rate increase to 140–150 within two to three minutes of exercise. No wonder they complained of fatigue.

I wanted to learn how to help these people; what interventions could decrease the frequency or intensity of their symptoms. What I found was information on the use of medications. Since most people were fairly young and did not want to take medications, I thought there must be other alternatives. I remember asking these people what they believed caused symptoms to improve or worsen. This was during the time of the initial reports on autonomic nervous system dysfunction in people with MVP. It wasn't until later that more information became available about this syndrome. From what people shared, and from information extrapolated from the literature, certain non-drug interventions became apparent.

Over the years, I carefully listened and reviewed literature. In talking with people with MVP, certain recurring themes became evident. One of these themes was how certain types of exercise reduced their symptoms. Why was that? Interestingly enough, I was unable to find any information in the literature on the effects of physical conditioning in people with symptomatic MVP. As a matter of fact, there were no research-based guidelines for exercise in this population, i.e., the type of exercise, how often, how much, *et cetera.*

During this time, one of my responsibilities was to develop and direct The Health Promotion and Rehabilitation Center. Our initial program was cardiac rehabilitation. We encouraged people with MVPS to exercise. Therefore, we had several of these persons at the Center. Since guidelines had not been established as to what exercise protocol was most appropriate, we used an exercise protocol similar to that used in a Phase II cardiac rehabilitation program. We attempted to group people with MVPS together, not only because their exercise tolerance was much lower, but because they could get to know others with similar complaints and compare their war stories. The people with MVP who were exercising at the Center reported noticeable decreases in their symptoms. This reduction in symptoms was usually greater than with the non-drug interventions alone. Why was that? Was it related to psychosocial, or physical aspects, or both?

I believe that in order for people to assume responsibility for their own health, they need guidance to assist themselves with symptom control. In order to give proper direction, appropriate guidelines are needed. These guidelines should have a sound basis. For instance, was the exercise protocol appropriate? Is three days a week enough? Is the type of exercise appropriate? These questions, along with others, were the basis of my PhD dissertation. The results were quite interesting. I must admit that initially I believed that most people would probably have to exercise more than three times a week to achieve a training effect that is usually seen after a 12-week period of exercise. The findings of the study, however, did not support my belief. I found that people had substantial improvement in their exercise capacity after exercising three times a week for a period of 12 weeks.

During the preliminary phase of the study, the idea for an MVP program was conceived. Thus, the Mitral Valve Prolapse Program of Cincinnati (MVPPC) was started. Although the program initially started as an educational-and-exercise program, it has grown to include diagnostic services, specialized testing, support groups, public seminars, counseling, and a quarterly newsletter. Through the many people we see at the MVPPC, I have the opportunity to gain more insight into this syndrome. The goal of this book is to share with you what others and I learned from working with people with MVPS, their families, and from what is published.

— *Kristine Scordo*

Understanding the
Mitral Valve Prolapse Syndrome

"I'm only 25 years old. How could I be having a heart attack?"

"I was given no explanation other than 'don't worry'."

"We would race to the hospital only to be sent home."

"I was beginning to believe I was crazy — it was all in my head."

"I feel like a second-class citizen. How come no one is taking this seriously?"

The story is all too familiar. First, you search for a diagnosis. After several visits with a physician and multiple tests, you're finally given a reason for the symptoms, and then told — don't worry. Now the questions begin. "What do I have? Mitral valve what? What does that mean? Will it get worse? Does my valve have to be replaced? Am I having a heart attack because I have chest pain? Will this affect my pregnancy? Is this common? How can I feel better?"

More than likely, you had similar thoughts and questions when you were first diagnosed with mitral-valve prolapse. Perhaps you still have a number of questions. Let me begin by telling you, you are not alone. You are among millions of people with MVP — or MVPers.

Mitral valve prolapse is a well-recognized, clinical entity with a reported prevalence of 4% to 18%. According to The Framingham Heart Study, 7.6% of women and 2.5% of men have MVP. Others report an incidence as high as 18% in women, and 12% in men. The wide range is due to gender, age, and ethnic background of the subjects, along with the use of different diagnostic criteria.

How many people with symptomatic mitral valve prolapse syndrome is unknown.

Mitral valve prolapse is believed to be inherited, with a greater expression of the MVP gene in females. Although people with MVP come in all shapes and sizes, there are physical features commonly associated with MVP. These include: pectus excavatum — depression of the breast bone, scoliosis — curvature of the spine, abnormally straight thoracic spine — straight back, arm span greater than height, unusual joint flexibility, and low body weight.

Mitral valve prolapse has been around for a long time. In fact, symptoms similar to MVP syndrome were traced to the sixteen hundreds. MVP has been known by a variety of names. These include: irritable heart, soldier's heart, the effort syndrome, Barlow's Syndrome, and DaCosta's Syndrome. British solders during the mid-eighteen hundreds noted symptoms of fatigue, palpitations, shortness of breath, chest pain and were unable to perform demanding physical tasks. This was a major cause of medical disability. Similar findings were noted during the Civil War, World War I and World War II.

William Osler, an eminent physician, noted the similarity between symptoms associated with irritable heart mentioned by others and those occurring in the general population, particularly in women. Some physicians believed the problem was not the heart, but one of a psychiatric nature. As technology advanced, so did the understanding of mitral valve prolapse. The 1980's saw the development of the classification of mitral valve prolapse into: Anatomic MVP and the MVP Syndrome.

Anatomic Mitral Valve Prolapse

Anatomic mitral valve prolapse is an abnormality of the mitral valve leaflets, or supporting chords, or both. These structures allow the leaflet(s) to prolapse — buckle back into the left atrium during the heart's contraction — ventricular systole. Anatomic mitral valve prolapse is usually associated with structural changes whereby: the valve can be described as floppy; the chords — supporting structure — may thin, thicken, or lengthen. The exact cause of these structural changes is theoretical and not clearly understood.

Several mechanisms can produce MVP. When the cause of the prolapse cannot be identified, it is described as *primary* mitral valve prolapse. When MVP is a consequence of other conditions, it is known as *secondary* mitral valve prolapse. One example of secondary mitral valve prolapse is prolapse caused by endocarditis — a bacterial infection of the valve. Please note that this book will discuss *primary* mitral valve prolapse

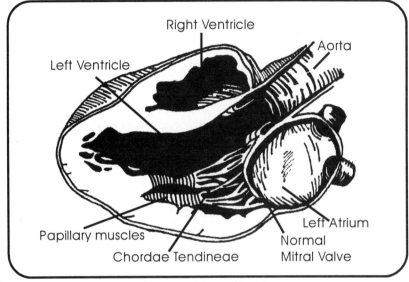

NORMAL MITRAL VALVE

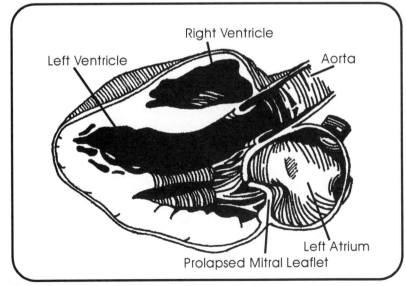

PROLAPSE OF THE MITRAL VALVE

Mitral Valve Prolapse Syndrome

Primary anatomic mitral valve prolapse is frequently associated with a constellation of symptoms. These symptoms are listed below. Individuals with one or more of these symptoms are referred to as having the mitral valve prolapse *syndrome* — MVPS. The term MVP syndrome refers to the occurrence of, or coexistence of, symptoms unexplainable on the basis of the valvular abnormality. *Thus, the symptoms associated with MVPS are not due to the valve itself.* They are believed to be based on various physiological changes. These are discussed later.

MITRAL VALVE PROLAPSE SYNDROME
COMMON SYMPTOMS

- Chest pain

- Fatigue

- Palpitations, extra heart beat

- Lightheadedness, dizziness

- Shortness of breath

- Anxiety and/or panic attacks

- Headaches

- Low exercise tolerance

- Mood swings

Characteristics of the Symptoms

Chest Pain

The chest pain associated with MVP presents itself in many ways. The pain may be brief in duration, or persist for hours. People describe the pain as sharp, heavy, shooting, sticking, or as pressure. At times it can be incapacitating, occurring repeatedly. Often the chest pain is atypical of angina — pain caused by narrowing or constriction in the coronary arteries. Sometimes, however, the pain mimics angina.

Many MVPers believe chest pains signal a heart attack. MVPS is not known to cause a heart attack. In general, severe narrowing and blockage of a coronary artery that supplies an area of heart muscle with blood causes a heart attack. This may lead to permanent damage of a portion of the heart muscle. MVPS neither narrows nor blocks coronary arteries, nor causes permanent damage to the heart muscle.

You ask, "How can I be sure the chest pain is not from coronary artery disease?" The answer to this relates to your original diagnosis. To first determine if heart disease is present, your physician considers your cardiovascular risk factors such as: age, sex, family history, blood lipid profile, smoking history, as well as your symptoms and results of diagnostic testing. Periodically, he follows up with testing such as an exercise stress test to reassure you the chest pain is not caused by coronary artery disease.

Fatigue

Fatigue is usually present to some degree. It may be episodic and severe, or relatively constant. Usually fatigue begets more fatigue — the less you do, the less you feel like doing. The cause of the fatigue may relate to blood volume changes noted with exercise, to a high resting heart rate, or to other physiological factors to be discussed shortly.

Palpitations, Extra Heart Beats, Forceful Heart Beat, Pounding Heart, Heart Flutter

People describe palpitations — extra beats — as a pounding sensation in their chest. Others say they feel a flip-flop or fluttering. Arrhythmias — disturbances in the heart rhythm — such as atrial extra beats (PACs), or premature ventricular extrasystoles (PVCs) can cause palpitations. While some people feel each beat, others do not notice them. Often, after extra beats, people have a sensation that their heart stopped for a few seconds.

Skipped or extra beats are very common among MVPers and the general public. Sometimes they occur following the use of caffeine, alcohol, tobacco, or certain medications. Other times, emotional stress may cause extra beats. Sometimes they happen for no apparent reason. In any case, these beats are relatively common, and should not be a cause for alarm. An explanation of the heart's electrical system may help to understand extra beats.

Each heartbeat normally starts in the right atrium. Here, a specialized group of cells called the sinus node — natural pacemaker — sets the pace for the heart's rhythm. From the sinus node, the electrical impulse spreads across the atria — the top part of the heart. This activity registers on the electrocardiogram (EKG) in the form of a blip, called the P wave. As the electrical impulse travels down the specialized conduction system to the ventricles, a QRS complex is generated.

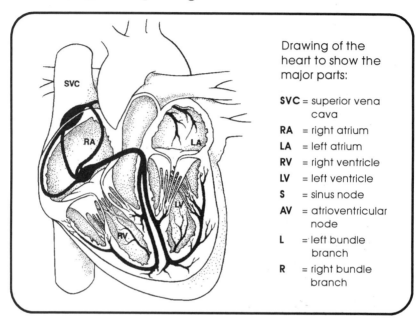

Drawing of the heart to show the major parts:

SVC = superior vena cava

RA = right atrium

LA = left atrium

RV = right ventricle

LV = left ventricle

S = sinus node

AV = atrioventricular node

L = left bundle branch

R = right bundle branch

ELECTRICAL ACTIVITY OF THE HEART

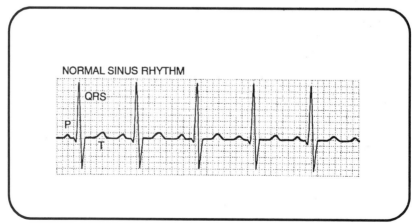

NORMAL SINUS RHYTHM

EKG TRACING

As the electrical signal travels through the heart, the heart contracts. First, the atria — top chambers — contract, pumping blood into the ventricles. A fraction of a second later, the ventricles — bottom chambers — contract, sending blood throughout the body. After each contraction, the heart relaxes for a brief moment. This relaxation produces the T wave on the EKG.

The heart normally contracts between 60 and 100 times per minute. Each contraction equals one heartbeat. This series of events occurs over 100,000 times a day. Alterations in the normal electrical sequence result in arrhythmias — disturbances in the heart rhythm.

There are many types of arrhythmias. Arrhythmias are identified by *where* they occur in the heart, and by *what* happens to the heart's rhythm when they occur. Arrhythmias sometimes originate in the atria or ventricles. They sometimes occur as a single beat or as repeated periods of very fast heartbeats. When a beat occurs early in the atria, it is known as a premature atrial beat or contraction. An atrial tachycardia occurs when a series of early atrial beats increase the heart rate. In paroxysmal tachycardia, repeated periods of very fast heartbeats begin and end suddenly.

TESTS FOR DETECTING ARRHYTHMIAS

- Resting Electrocardiogram: While at rest, disks or electrodes are placed on the chest, arms, and legs and a recording taken.

- Graded Exercise Stress Test: Exercise on a treadmill machine or bicycle while connected to the EKG machine.

- 24-hour Holter Monitor: Ambulatory monitor that records the EKG over a period of 24 hours.

- Transtelephone or Event Monitor: A monitoring device worn from several days to several weeks. When the arrhythmia is felt, it is transmitted over the phone and the EKG recorded, or stored in the monitor's memory and transmitted at a later time.

- Electrophysiologic Study: An invasive test that involves cardiac catheterization. Thin, flexible tubes — catheters — are placed in an arm or leg vein and advanced to the heart. This allows for special recordings to be made.

Arrhythmias can be detected by listening to the heart with a stethoscope. An arrhythmia may not be present, however, at the time of the examination. Therefore, other tests are needed to detect the arrhythmia. The type of test depends on how often the arrhythmia occurs, and in what setting. For example, if activity brings on the arrhythmia, a graded exercise stress test is indicated. Otherwise, if the arrhythmia occurs infrequently, an event monitor would be appropriate.

Premature ventricular contractions are common in MVPers. PVCs originate from an electrical signal in the ventricles, and occur prematurely in the cardiac cycle. Depending upon the prematurity of the PVC, it may not allow the heart enough time to fill with blood. This causes an ineffective contraction. Therefore, the heart doesn't pump its full requirement of blood. After the premature ventricular beat, sometimes a sensation occurs that the heart stopped. To understand this sensation, think of the heart as a large rubber band. The greater you stretch the rubber band, the harder it springs back. When a beat is premature and the heart doesn't have adequate time to fill with blood, the rubber band — heart muscle — stretches a little and doesn't bounce back as much. The heart, therefore, doesn't do the same amount of work, or pump the same amount of blood. If you take your pulse, you don't feel the premature beat.

Next, the heart pauses — a compensatory pause — to compensate for the prematurity of PVC. This pause causes the sensation that the heart has stopped. It allows the heart more time to fill with blood. Therefore, the rubber band stretches farther, and the heart's contraction becomes more forceful — the "flip-flop" feeling. It is the beat *after* the extra beat that most people feel.

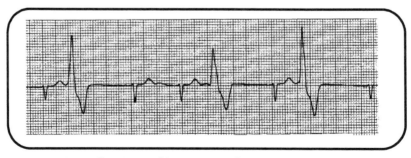

PREMATURE VENTRICULAR CONTRACTIONS

When people describe palpitations, or a forceful heart beat, arrhythmias may not be noted. What may be felt is sinus tachycardia — a speeding up of the natural heart beat. Everyday, almost everyone has periods when his rate exceeds 100 beats per minute. Exercise, anxiety, and secret rendezvous with your lover naturally increase your heart rate. Too, when you are out of shape — deconditioned — and running up a flight of stairs, your heart rapidly pounds.

There is often a discordance between the EKG and the person's *sensations* of extra beats or *sensations* of a pounding heart. During 24-hour Holter monitor recordings, MVPers record palpitations in the diary, and believe they have an arrhythmia. When the EKG tracings are reviewed, only sinus tachycardia is noted.

TYPES OF ARRHYTHMIAS

- Sinus tachycardia: A speeding up of the natural pacemaker of the heart to rates over 100 beats per minute.

- Sinus bradycardia: A slowing down of the natural pacemaker of the heart to rates less than 60 beats per minute.

- Premature atrial contraction: A beat that occurs early in the atria and causes the heart to beat prematurely.

- Paroxysmal supraventricular tachycardia (PSVT): A series of repeated beats that originate above the ventricles and speed up the heart rate. Usually PSVT begins and ends suddenly.

- Atrial fibrillation: Electrical signals in the atria fire multiple electrical impulses. A fraction of these impulses make their way down to the ventricles in an irregular fashion. This makes the pulse rate very irregular.

- Premature ventricular contraction — PVC: An electrical signal from the ventricles that causes the heart to beat before the next regular heartbeat.

- Ventricular tachycardia: Three or more premature ventricular contractions that occur together.

- Ventricular fibrillation: Electrical signals are fired from the ventricles in a very fast and chaotic manner. This causes the heart to lose its ability to pump blood.

Lightheadedness, Dizziness

Lightheadedness, dizziness, or both can occur when first standing up. This feeling is usually associated with a sensation of a forceful heart beat or palpitations. These symptoms may be related to decreased intravascular volume and metabolic neuroendocrine abnormalities.

Shortness of Breath

This is usually described as the inability to take in a deep breath. It may occur at rest or with activity. The shortness of breath has not been found to be related to cardiac — heart, or pulmonary — lung abnormalities.

Anxiety and/or Panic Attacks

Although the relationship is not clear, many MVPers suffer from anxiety or panic attacks. The symptoms described are more consistent with panic disorder, the anxiety disorder studied most often in MVP patients. People have recurrent, spontaneous anxiety attacks that consist of various combinations of symptoms similar to some MVPS symptoms. These symptoms include: fatigue, fainting, dizziness, chest pain, lightheadedness, rapid heartbeat, heart palpitations, and shortness of breath.

The degree and mechanism of association between MVPS and anxiety disorders remains unclear. While some believe the symptoms cause anxiety attacks, others believe extraneous factors trigger attacks. They may occur anywhere, at anytime, even in the middle of the night. Whenever anxiety attacks do occur, they are frightening.

Headaches

Headaches sometimes occur in the form of migraines and are accompanied by nausea and blurred vision. Some people describe their headaches as nagging or dull.

Other Symptoms

MVPers report other symptoms. Common ones include:

- Chronically cold hands and feet
- Gastrointestinal — stomach — disturbances
- Problems with memory or a feeling of fogginess
- Inability to concentrate
- Mood swings
- Problems sleeping
- Numbness or tingling of the arms or legs
- Arm, back, or shoulder discomfort
- Difficulty swallowing
- Lump in the throat

Frequently, these symptoms are frightening, discomforting, frustrating, annoying, and incapacitating. Certainly, they affect one's life style.

Expect symptoms to be more intense during emotional stress, when you are overly tired, after unaccustomed physical activities, during menopause, or during menstruation. It is not unusual for the symptoms to disappear spontaneously for months — even years — and reappear again.

The table on page 12 lists factors that increase the intensity or frequency of MVPS symptoms. Data collected at the Mitral Valve Prolapse Program of Cincinnati (MVPPC), along with responses to the questionnaire in the first edition of *Taking Control* were used to compile the list.

Symptoms begin at any age. Most people, however, notice symptoms between the ages of 20 to 30. The exact cause likely relates to several factors and remains unclear. Often, MVPers who have been without symptoms, become symptomatic after an illness, injury, pregnancy, or emotional stress such as a divorce. While symptoms occur more in females, many also occur in male MVPers. Frequently, chest pain, palpitations, fatigue, or anxiety attacks initially prompt them to seek medical help.

Many people with MVPS believe the more symptoms they have, the more severe is the prolapse — buckling back of the valve. This is *not* the case. In the mitral valve prolapse syndrome, there is no correlation between the degree of prolapse and the severity of the symptoms.

FACTORS THAT CAN INCREASE THE INTENSITY OR FREQUENCY OF MVPS SYMPTOMS

- Emotional stress

- Excessive fatigue

- Unaccustomed physical activity

- Being anxious or nervous

- Caffeine

- Medicines with stimulants

- Sweets

- Being in a hot, dry environment

- Dehydration

- Flu, cold, or other illnesses

- Lack of sleep

- Alcohol

- Smoking

- Skipping meals

- Rushing around

- Lying on the left or right side

- Menses

- Menopause

Metabolic-neuroendocrine Abnormalities in MVPS

Research studies support the belief that certain physiological abnormalities may be responsible for MVPS symptoms. Not *everyone's* symptoms, however, are explained by these physiological alterations. The presence, degree, and type of involvement of the various physiological systems sometimes vary.

These physiological abnormalities include: autonomic nervous system dysfunction, decreased intravascular blood volume, and renin-aldosterone regulation abnormality. These systems are-interrelated but separately discussed.

Autonomic Nervous System Dysfunction

The body is under the constant control of the CNS — the central nervous system. This system is essential for our sense of well-being and our normal daily performance. The central nervous system controls and regulates in order to provide both stability and rapid, adaptive change to internal and external factors. Also, the central nervous system provides physiological, anticipatory adjustments. In other words, while certain body responses are under voluntary control, others are under involuntary control. For example, when you exercise your heart rate normally increases to meet the demands of your body — an involuntary response. This response is controlled by the *Autonomic Nervous System* — involuntary part of the CNS.

Two divisions comprise the autonomic nervous system: the parasympathetic system — the decelerator, and the sympathetic system — the accelerator. In general, parasympathetic responses dominate when we are quiet, relaxed or asleep, and sympathetic responses dominate when we are alert, excited, or engaged in muscular exercise. Note the following example that explains how these systems work.

You peacefully drive down the highway. Suddenly a MACK truck heads toward you. Your sympathetic nervous system — the accelerator — goes into action. It releases adrenalin. Your heart rate increases; your pupils dilate; and the blood supply to your muscles increases. Instantly, you have better braking action and can see better. You successfully avoid the truck. Now, to slow things down, the parasympathetic nervous system — the decelerator — takes over. It releases acetylcholine — a chemical substance and you are-ready to deal with the runaway army tank.

Catecholamines are the chemical substances the sympathetic nervous system releases. Two major catecholamines are epinephrine — adrenalin, and norepinephrine. When these substances are released, they interact with cells in the blood vessels and in various organs. The part of the cell that responds to these chemicals is the receptor. A receptor is believed to be a site on the cell's surface where chemicals attach and initiate specific cellular processes.

Think of these receptors and chemicals as locks and keys — the lock is the receptor, and the chemical is the key. Whenever any key is turned, it determines a certain response. For example, epinephrine — depending upon which receptors are activated — causes blood vessels in skeletal muscle to narrow — vasocon-striction, or to enlarge — vasodilatation. Interaction of these chemicals with cells in the heart's electrical pacemaker, increase the heart rate.

Instability, or imbalance, results when either the sympathetic system or the parasympathetic system are too active. This imbalance is referred to as *dysautonomia* — or autonomic dysfunction. People with MVPS sometimes have higher levels of catecholamines, alterations in catecholamine regulation, hypersensitivity to catecholamine stimulation and heightened parasympathetic responses. In other words, there is an increased number of locks, or keys, or both. These findings are believed to be responsible for a number of MVPS symptoms.

Dysautonomia — imbalance in the autonomic nervous system — is noted in people who have all the classic symptoms of MVPS, but have no objective findings of mitral valve prolapse. In other words, the person has no extra heart sounds or evidence of MVP on the echocardiogram. Their symptoms, however, are controllable with the non-drug treatments discussed in Chapter 3.

Renin-Aldosterone Regulation Abnormality

Research studies indicate some individuals with MVPS have alterations in how the body regulates water and sodium — salt, or the renin-aldosterone regulating system.

Aldosterone is the principal sodium-retaining steroid hormone — chemical substance. It maintains normal fluid balance and circulatory blood volume — fluid contained within the circulatory system. Normally, when blood volume decreases, as occurs with dehydration, the sympathetic nervous system activates and a special enzyme — renin — secretes. This results in the release of aldosterone. Aldosterone causes sodium to be reabsorbed by the kidney and fluid to be retained. When blood volume is restored, renin secretion is suppressed.

In MVPS, there may be an abnormality in the regulation of this system. Studies show that after volume depletion caused by taking diuretics — water pills, renin activity and aldosterone release are reduced. Furthermore, renin activity is inappropriately low for the decreased circulating blood volume noted in people with MVPS.

Imagine this system as Larry-the-lock controller on a dam. When the water level gets low — decreased circulating blood volume — Larry turns the wheel and closes the gates. The closed gates hold the water back, and cause a higher water level. Now, Larry becomes tired and doesn't close the wheel. What happens? The gates stay open, and the water level stays low. Likewise, this sometimes happens in MVPS — Larry lacks the energy to close the gates all the way.

Decreased Intravascular Volume

The volume of blood contained within the circulatory system is called the intravascular volume. It contains both plasma and the cellular elements of the blood. This blood volume is regulated through an intricate feedback mechanism. The integrity of this feedback mechanism is maintained by the kidneys, which regulate the blood volume either through an increase or decrease in urine excretion.

Studies indicate that people with MVPS sometimes have decreased plasma and intravascular volumes, which may be partly responsible for the lightheadedness, dizziness, and a forceful heart beat noted when first standing up.

Normally, whenever you stand from a lying position, cardiac output — amount of blood the heart pumps in a minute — increases. In some MVPers, however, cardiac output decreases when they first stand up. The decrease in cardiac output, along with a decrease in blood pressure and an increase in heart rate, cause feelings of lightheadedness, dizziness, and forceful heart pounding.

Likewise, this reduction in cardiac output — noted upon standing — may also continue during exercise. Coupled with the relatively high resting heart rate, it offers an explanation for the exercise intolerance and fatigue noted with MVPS.

The variations in intravascular volume and reduced renin aldosterone activity help explain why some MVPers are very susceptible to volume depletion. These people note their symptoms worsen after taking water pills or during crash dieting. Both cause water loss.

Magnesium Deficiency

Magnesium is an essential mineral required for multiple body functions. It is the fourth most common cation in the body and the second most common — after potassium — cation in cells.

More than 300 enzymatic reactions depend on magnesium. This mineral affects the contractility of muscles, affects nerve conduction, and affects electrolyte balance. In the cardiovascular system magnesium influences both cardiac electrical and mechanical properties, and reactivity of blood vessels.

The adult human body contains approximately 21 to 28 grams of magnesium. Approximately 60% of body magnesium is in the bone, 35% is found in the muscle, and 1% is found in the extracellular — outside the cell — fluid compartment.

Most magnesium is *intra*cellular — inside the body cells. Conversely, *extra*cellular means outside the body cells. Therefore, a routine serum, or extracellular blood test inaccurately reflects magnesium concentration within the body cells.

For example, muscle levels of magnesium may be low, but serum levels are normal. The introduction of special blood tests, such as atomic absorption spectroscopy (RBC Mg), allows for more-accurate determination of total *intra*cellular magnesium.

Although controversial, evidence indicates that many features of MVP syndrome may be attributed to the physiologic effects of magnesium deficiency. Some people with MVPS have low blood levels of magnesium, particularly those with muscle cramps and migraines — two symptoms of magnesium deficiency. Other symptoms of magnesium deficiency include: muscular weakness, lethargy, nausea, tremors, cardiac arrhythmias, and psychiatric abnormalities such as anxiety, depression or nervous-hyperexcitability.

Magnesium deficiency can be due to a reduced intake, reduced absorption, increased excretion or redistribution of magnesium within the body. Large-scale dietary surveys reveal the dietary intake of magnesium of most Americans falls below the recommended dietary allowance. Foods highest in magnesium — legumes, whole grains, and dark green leafy vegetables — are not major constituents of the average American diet. Also, reduced intake of magnesium occurs with dieting. Reduced absorption can occur with high saturated fat diets, or with the intake of substances such as dietary phosphates — very high in some sodas. Increased excretion can be caused by alcohol ingestion, diuretics — water pills, or excess sugar intake. Redistribution of magnesium occurs when levels of catecholamines are increased, as seen during psychological and physical stress. All of these factors increase magnesium requirements.

Diagnosing Mitral Valve Prolapse

Being diagnosed with MVP can be problematic. Some of the symptoms associated with MVPS may be present in a variety of other clinical conditions. Therefore, people often say MVP was not their initial diagnosis. See Chapter 2. Many MVPers consulted several physicians and received conflicting diagnoses as listed below:

- Hypoglycemia — low blood sugar
- Chronic fatigue syndrome
- Hypothyroidism; hyperthyroidism
- Meniere's disease — inner ear problem
- Anxiety disorder
- Multiple sclerosis
- Fibromyalgia
- Esophagitis

In making the diagnosis of MVP, the physician considers a variety of factors. These include your present symptoms, past history, family history, results of the physical examination and diagnostic tests.

A key factor in diagnosing mitral valve prolapse is auscultation — listening — of the heart. The presence of a click with or without a systolic murmur is characteristic of MVP. The click is an extra heart sound caused by the tensing of the chords that facilitate the opening and closing of the valve. A systolic murmur is a sound that occurs during the heart's contraction when a small amount of blood flows backward — through a partially opened mitral valve — into the left atrium.

Changes in posture may alter the characteristics of the click and murmur. Your physician, therefore, may listen to your heart when you are: squatting, standing, lying down, or lying on your left side. MVP is a very dynamic syndrome, however, and the click or murmur may not always be heard. People commonly say, "Sometimes my physician hears the click, and sometimes he doesn't." Also, if you take beta blockers or tranquilizers, or are well hydrated, the click or murmur — or both — may be inaudible.

**MOST COMMON SYMPTOMS
FOR SEEKING ASSISTANCE OF A PHYSICIAN***

- Palpitations, extra beats, irregular heartbeat, pounding heart, racing heart, skipped beats, rapid pulse, heart fluttering

- Chest pain, chest tightness

- Lightheadedness, dizziness, almost passing out

- Fatigue, weakness

- Anxiety/panic attacks

- Shortness of breath

- Headaches

*Data from *Taking Control* questionnaire.

The echocardiogram can be used to confirm the diagnosis. This ultrasound examination of the heart consists of an M-mode — or ice-pick view — of the heart along with a two dimensional — 2D — view. This test gives information about the mitral valve, the other valves, the thickness of the walls of the heart, the size of the heart's chambers, and how well the heart contracts. Color Doppler shows the presence and degree of mitral regurgitation — or backward blood flow. It is not uncommon to have MVP, but not see it on the echocardiogram. This is known as a false-negative reading. Usually, if MVP shows on the echo, it continues to show in future studies.

To screen for possible coronary artery disease, a graded exercise stress test is done. Prior to the start of a stress test, the technician places foam-filled disks on your chest. The disks connect to wires. The wires connect to a heart monitor. The monitor records your heart's electrical activity. As you walk on the treadmill, the speed and grade — height — of the treadmill increase at specified times. (A bicycle may be used in place of the treadmill.) The technician monitors your blood pressure before, during, and after the test. The test provides information about your level of cardiovascular fitness, your blood pressure response to exercise, and any exercise-induced abnormalities in heart rhythm. Also, this test may show EKG changes that *suggest* ischemia — lack of oxygen to a portion of the heart muscle. This may, however, be a false-positive result.

At times, MVPers have false-positive exercise stress tests that occur with or without chest pain. In other words, there are changes on the EKG similar to that seen with ischemic coronary artery disease; but, the person does not have heart coronary artery disease. In this situation, a test that combines a graded exercise stress test with the injection of a radioisotope provides further diagnostic information. Exercise Tc^{99m}Cardiolite or Thallium-201 are examples.

When these radioisotopes are injected, they normally distribute throughout the heart muscle. The amount of the isotope the heart muscle takes up is directly related to its blood flow. If a coronary artery is narrowed or blocked, the isotope doesn't distribute to the area supplied by this artery. Therefore, when pictures of the heart are taken, a cold spot or dark area shows on the film. At a later time, the pictures are repeated. If the cold spot no longer shows, it suggests a narrowing of a coronary artery. If the cold spot remains, it suggests a previous heart attack.

Sometimes, a heart catheterization may be needed This involves injecting small amounts of dye into the coronary arteries via a catheter or small hollow tube. A physician usually recommends this for any number of reasons. Is the person over 40? Does he have a strong family history of heart disease or other cardiac risk factors? Are there suspicious symptoms of coronary artery disease? Was the exercise nuclear study abnormal?

After you have been diagnosed with MVP, the follow-up with your physician is similar to others without MVP, i.e., annual physical examination. Some physicians recommend repeat echocardiograms every few years to note changes in the mitral valve structure, the chamber sizes, the wall thickness, and the heart muscle's contractions. Consult your physician if your symptoms change, or if you are unsure if they relate to MVPS.

The presence and degree of dysautonomia is determined by autonomic testing. This involves the use of noninvasive, cardiovascular reflex tests. A noninvasive test does not require any needle punctures, incisions, or insertion of instruments. These reflex tests include:

1. The heart rate response to a simulated Valsalva maneuver — with your nose closed, blowing into a mouthpiece at a certain pressure

2. Deep breathing

3. Blood pressure and heart rate responses to standing — or with head up on a tilt table

4. Sustained handgrip — holding a special handgrip device. There are normal responses to these tests. Sometimes the test is repeated and results compared to determine the efficacy of certain treatment interventions. Furthermore, your level of plasma catecholamines can be determined. This blood test measures levels of epinephrine and norepinephrine.

SUMMARY

MVPS — a common clinical condition — affects millions of people. Only within the past few years have researchers identified a physiological basis for its symptoms.

Previously — as letters from MVPers show — many endured one misdiagnosis after another till some truly believed, "It's all in my head."

Although definitive words on methods for long-term treatment of MVPS await further research, don't give up. Follow the recommendations discussed in this book. Use this knowledge to change the quality of your life. TAKE CONTROL.

SELECTED REFERENCES

Bashore, T., Grines , C., Utlak, D., Boudoulas, J., & Wooley, C. 1985. "Mitral valve prolapse: Postural exercise response reflects a volume disorder." *Journal of the American College of Cardiology*. **5:** 504 (abstr).

Boudoulas, J. 1992. "Mitral valve prolapse: Etiology, clinical presentation and neuroendocrine function." *Journal Heart Valve Disease*. **1:** 175–188.

Boudoulas, J. & Wooley, C. 1988. "Mitral valve prolapse: Clinical presentation and diagnostic evaluation." In: *Mitral Valve Prolapse and the Mitral Valve Prolapse Syndrome* (H. Boudoulas & C. Wooley, Eds.). Futura Publ. Co., Inc. New York. 299–330.

Coghlan, H. & Natello, G. 1991. "Erythrocyte magnesium in symptomatic patients with primary mitral valve prolapse: Relationship to symptoms, mitral leaflet thickness, joint hypermobility and autonomic regulation." *Magnesium Trace Element*. **92:** 205–214.

Coghlan, H., Phares, P., Cowley, M., Copley, D., & James, T. 1979. "Dysautonomia in mitral valve prolapse." *American Journal of Medicine*. **67:** 236–244.

Elin, R. 1988. "Magnesium metabolism in health and disease." *Disease of the Month*. 34: 161–219.

Ewing, D. 1988. "Recent advances in the non-invasive investigation of diabetic autonomic neuropathy." In: *Autonomic Failure: A Textbook of Clinical Disorders of the Autonomic Nervous System* (R. Bannister, Ed.). Oxford University Press. Oxford. 667–689

Fontana, M., Wooley, C., Leighton, R., & Lewis, R. 1975. "Postural changes in left ventricular andmitral valvular dynamics in the systolic click-late systolic murmur syndrome." *Circulation*. **51:** 165–173.

Gaffney, F. & Blomqvist, C. 1988. "Mitral valve prolapse and autonomic nervous system dysfunction: A pathophysiological link." In: *Mitral Valve Prolapse and the Mitral Valve Prolapse Syndrome* (H. Boudoulas & C. Wooley, Eds.). Futura Publ. Co., Inc. New York. 427–443.

Galland, L., Baker, S., & McLellan, R. 1986. "Magnesium deficiency in the pathogenesis of mitral valve prolapse." *Magnesium*. **5:** 165–174.

Halpern, M. & Durlach, J. (Eds.) 1985. "Magnesium deficiency: Physiopathology and treatment implications." First European congress on Magnesium, Lisbon, October 6–8, 1983. Karger. New York.

Jeresaty, R. 1979. *Mitral Valve Prolapse*. Raven Press. New York.

Kolibash, A. 1988. "Natural history of mitral valve prolapse." In: *Mitral Valve Prolapse and the Mitral Valve Prolapse Syndrome.* (H. Boudoulas & C. Wooley, Eds.) Futura Publ. Co., Inc. New York. 257–274.

Rude, R. 1989. "Physiology of magnesium metabolism and the important role of magnesium in potassium deficiency." *American Journal of Cardiology*. **63:** 31G–43G.

Seeing, M. 1989. "Cardiovascular consequences of magnesium deficiency and loss: Pathogenesis, prevalence and manifestations magnesium and chloride loss in refractory potassium repletion." *American Journal of Cardiology*. **63:** 4G–22G.

2

People with MVPS
Share Their Experiences

"The universe is made of stories, not of atoms."
(Rukeyser, 1980)

According to your many letters and responses to the questionnaire in the first edition of *Taking Control*, this chapter was the most popular. Comments such as these were common. "I'm so glad to hear I'm not alone. " "That sounds just like me." "I really enjoyed reading what others did to control their symptoms."

In the fall of 1992, because of these comments the feature "Tell It Like It Is" began in Network, the newsletter of The MVP Program of Cincinnati. This column encouraged people to share their experiences. Letters poured in from all of the world, and we continue to receive dozens of letters weekly.

Stories range from those who, on the first visit, were correctly diagnosed with MVPS to those who, after *dozens* of visits to various physicians were diagnosed with MVPS. Many say their symptoms interfere with activities of daily living, with family relations, and with work relations. Frequently, individuals share fears experienced before they were correctly diagnosed — fears of not knowing what was going on and why they had symptoms. Some were told, "It's all in you head," and believed they were going crazy. Others became unsettled when told, "You have MVP and chest pain ... don't worry about it."

As you read the following accounts from real people with MVPS, you may identify with certain aspects of their stories. Some of these individuals either completed the program or attended the educational seminars — others didn't. Some were diagnosed recently — others were diagnosed years ago. In several of the following accounts, note two recurring themes: initial distress, noted prior to diagnosis, and later comfortableness, noted after diagnosis and explanations.

Kathy

"Living with MVPS has not been easy for me or for those around me, but I learned how to control it and how to live a normal life.

"As I grew up, I complained about my heart doing flip-flops, speeding up, and then slowing down for no apparent reason. Since no one worried about this, I did not. I never imagined what was to follow. I will never forget the night I woke up suddenly with terrible chest pains, shortness of breath, and an unnerving fear that I was dying. "I'm only 25 years old," I said. "How could I be having a heart attack?"

> I'm only 25 years old. How could I be having a heart attack?

"I refused to go back to sleep — afraid I would never awaken. This was the start of endless symptoms: chest pains, headaches, heart palpitations, panic attacks, shortness of breath, fatigue, dizziness, and even fainting.

"I went to a physician who diagnosed MVP. He, however, ran additional tests that ruled out problems with similar symptoms. These tests came back negative, and the echocardiogram confirmed his diagnosis. Now, I had a name for my symptoms — MVP — and a prescription for a beta blocker supposed to alleviate my symptoms, or so I thought. Other than, "Do not worry. There is nothing wrong with you," I received no further information.

> Other than, "Do not worry," I was given no explanations.

"Things worsened. I experienced symptoms daily that affected me, as well as those around me. Three or four times I went to the emergency room for fainting spells only to be told there was nothing life threatening. One physician said, 'Everything is in your head. You cause your own symptoms.'

"How could this be? I was miserable. Out of fear that something might happen, I avoided grocery stores and restaurants. I needed help. I needed to know more about mitral valve prolapse. About that time a co-worker told me about an advertisement on the radio for a seminar on MVP. Now, my life began to look up. Through seminars, and later on through support group meetings I learned how to deal with my MVPS. I now understand what MVP is and why things happen. I no longer fear that I am going to die.

"The greatest help to me was listening to others with MVP and knowing that I was not alone — we shared the same symptoms and fears. I learned how to control my symptoms without drugs. I ride an exercise bike regularly. I eliminate caffeine from my diet, increase my fluid intake, and use salt freely. In the past six months, I've had no severe symptoms. My life is becoming normal."

What follows is an account from Kathy's husband, Karl.

"My wife, Kathy, first experienced symptoms associated with MVP only about 10–12 months ago. My early reactions, therefore, are relatively fixed in my mind. In the past several months, I went through a cycle that began with fear, then disbelief, relief, annoyance, and finally understanding and adaptation. Let me explain.

"Kathy often commented in the past that her heart flip-flopped or sped up for no apparent reason. This never bothered either of us till one night she awakened with a full-blown panic attack: chest pains, shortness of breath — the works. This attack eventually passed. Then, when the symptoms recurred, I sensed that something was seriously wrong, but I tried not to let on. After two or three trips to the emergency room, however, I couldn't hide my feelings.

"After four or five weeks of severe symptoms, Kathy was diagnosed with MVP. When I learned this was not life threatening, my first reaction was disbelief. How could something that created such havoc *not* be life threatening? In fact, we even sought other physicians' opinions.

"Eventually, relief set in. I was convinced things were going to be all right. It was very comforting to have two physicians agree that it was MVP, and it could be controlled.

"My next stage — annoyance — is hard for me to discuss. I actually felt annoyed with my wife. After all Kathy had been through, I could not understand why she still felt symptoms, still had panic attacks, and still felt lethargic. I wanted to get on with our lives.

"We began to attend seminars and group sessions with other MVP patients. Now, I better understand what Kathy went through. I also understand how important it is for me to be supportive. Since we made some changes and adapted to living with MVP, we both know it is going to be all right."

Fred — *another husband's point of view*

"Husbands and boyfriends also need to become both educated and empathetic about MVPS. Unfortunately, my wife's symptoms sometimes negatively affect our relationship. For example, we forgo wonderful activities together, afraid that she may end up in the emergency room with palpitations or a panic attack. Furthermore, her medications cause fatigue and suppress both her emotions and her enthusiasm. Together, the syndrome and the drugs inhibit her spontaneity.

"I am devoted to my wife and want to do things as a couple. I feel, however, that life is leaving us behind. We are almost forty, slim, fit, and athletic but, we act as if we're over the hill. Although I surf, run, and work out with friends, I want to be with *her*. If I could convince her that an active life-style wouldn't hurt, it would be great.

"At times I feel she ignores me or pushes me aside. She bonds with other people with MVP for support. I want her to bond with me. To other spouses I say, 'Be informed; be supportive; and be optimistic. Repeatedly tell her she is OK. Don't put your life on hold.' "

Debbie

"I am not sure exactly when my symptoms began. During my teen-age years, however, I remember a pounding heart for which I took tranquilizers. I was extremely nervous, anxious, and bothered by a lump in my throat.

"About 10 years ago, at the age of 37, my symptoms surfaced and started to control me. I felt I was having a heart attack and was going to die. I had anxiety, pounding heart, palpitations, chest pains, and a fast heart rate. Many times I experienced a tightening feeling in my chest and became scared. I paced the floor; I stretched; I did anything to get rid of the symptoms.

I knew it wasn't all in my head.

"During that time — on Christmas Eve in 1983, in our presence my father-in-law had a stroke and was taken to the hospital. That night my heart raced, and I experienced chest pain. As a result, I went to see a general practitioner — my first mistake. I tried to share symptoms and relate my family history. He stopped me from telling him anything and examined me. 'There is nothing wrong with you; calm down,' he said. I tried to believe him, but the symptoms were there: the pounding heart, palpitations, chest pain, pain in my arm and jaw that didn't stop. I knew it wasn't all in my head.

"Next, I called my father-in-law's cardiologist, a knowledge-able, soft-spoken man. He said it sounded like MVP. I had an echocardiogram and Holter monitor done. He said I had MVP, shouldn't worry, that I wasn't going to die. Then, he started me on Inderal. I have been on medication since, and take Ativan when I need it. Over the years whenever my symptoms worsened, he increased my medications.

"I believe MVP controls my life at times. I try not to let it bother me, but sometimes it does. I am grateful for the influx of informa-tion on the subject and believe education is the key. How well I remember when I first went on medication. My sister-in-law said, 'Why are *you* under stress? *You* don't work.' I'll never forget it. Just because I wasn't working full time, I shouldn't have stress.

"I don't think my husband understands the impact MVP has had on me. I tried to explain it, but to a person who has never experienced it, I think it is hard to understand. Also, I have never been hospitalized for this or gone to the emergency room. He has never witnessed my having a problem so severe that I am hospi-talized.

"What I have read, and now that MVPS is being recognized has helped. Although I still have my moments, it certainly is not like the beginning.

"My 23-year-old son has been diagnosed with MVP. He has chest pain occasionally, but he's never been on medication."

Diana

"I am now 60. Until a year ago when I discovered the MVP pro-gram, I battled the unknown and survived the trauma of many misdiagnoses. I lived with severe panic attacks, sought profes-sional help, and endured all the bizarre symptoms mentioned in *Taking Control.*

> ... I am now 60 ... I battled the unknown and survived the trauma of every misdiagnosis ...

"Twenty years ago, after my husband's death, my life changed. Fear was my constant com-panion. I white knuckled my way through grad-uate school and into a new career. Family, friends, and physicians thought I imagined symptoms. As a result, I found myself in isola-tion.

"After a self diagnosis of anxiety, I used relaxation techniques, meditation, and drank calming herbs and teas. This lessened my symptoms.

"I enrolled in college — a challenge. I experienced dizziness, fatigue, shortness of breath, and was plagued with chronic shoulder pain. The desire to be thinner meant crash diets. Rather than meals, I drank tea or coffee. My full class schedule and new diet equaled trouble.

"Following college, during the first year of marriage, I worked 14 hours a day, and continued dieting. My symptoms became unbearable. Cardiologists at my husband's medical school diagnosed a heart murmur. They said to curtail all activity. The future looked bleak.

"My mother, not satisfied with the diagnosis, insisted I go to my hometown hospital. After a 24-hour monitor and an echocardiogram, I was diagnosed with MVP. I received information about penicillin use for dental procedures and surgery, and was instructed to resume my normal activities.

"The symptoms continued. At the request of physician friends, I continued to undergo testing. Diagnoses included: hypoglycemia, asthma, hiatal hernia and more. I took medications and suffered side effects. No one connected the symptoms with MVP.

"Now, with the help of the book and newsletters, I learned to take control. I noticed a tremendous difference when I followed the guidelines for diet, water intake, salt, caffeine, and chocolate. I read letters from others with MVP and feel reassured. I find the 'Top Ten List' helpful in reducing my anxiety — I refer to it several times a week. My symptoms along with my stress are alleviated by drinking calming herbs. My favorites contain valerian, passiflora, celery seed, catnip, hops, and orange peel."

Donna

"In the summer of 1990, I experienced dizzy spells and feelings of lightheadedness once or twice a week for brief moments. I blamed the summer heat and didn't believe the spells were serious. The dizzy spells lasted three to four weeks. Once they were gone, I didn't give them a second thought. In late November of 1990, the lightheadedness returned, and I experienced nervousness. My hands shook and my legs felt like lead. Because I didn't feel stressed I couldn't understand why I experienced unusual symptoms. I also experienced severe nasal congestion and stuffiness. I thought I was getting the flu or a bad cold.

"Nonprescription decongestants did nothing and made me feel worse. By early December, the symptoms increased in intensity and in frequency. The dizziness progressed. Whenever I walked or stood up from a sitting position, I felt as if I were riding on a fast elevator. I had extreme pain deep inside the middle area of my sinuses. I experienced rapid heartbeat, chest pains, and shortness of breath. I figured this bad case of the flu was out of hand and went to the emergency room. The attending physician could not explain the rapid heartbeat and diagnosed me with sinusitis. He prescribed an antihistamine and decongestant that gave me no relief.

"On the third day after drinking a half cup of coffee with my medication, my heart rate suddenly increased, and I couldn't breathe. I knew I was having a heart attack! Paramedics took me to the emergency room. The EKG, chest X-ray, and blood work were normal. The physician said, 'The flu is in your head. Go home. Don't drink any liquids or take medication with stimulants.'

"A week later, a family practice physician at my HMO also diagnosed me with sinusitis and prescribed mild medication. Nothing alleviated the dizziness, chest pains, or rapid heartbeats.

"Next, I was referred to an ear, nose, and throat specialist. He conducted various tests and said, 'You don't have sinusitis. It's possible you have mitral valve prolapse.' Three weeks passed. Then, an echocardiogram showed I did have MVP. No one explained this condition, and I was not able to speak with a cardiologist. The technicians told me that dizziness is not associated with MVP.

"I persisted with the validity of my symptoms and a CAT scan and Holter monitor were ordered. This physician said the dizziness was due to stress in my life. The CAT scan results were normal. The holter monitor revealed a fast heartbeat. My physician prescribed Inderal for the rapid beats and Antivert for the dizziness. Although the Inderal helped the rapid heartbeat and chest pains, it made me very tired. I could barely function. It also affected my breathing. The Antivert helped the dizziness.

> ... I have MVP. However, no one explained what this is.

"Again, I switched physicians and HMO's. I went through the entire process of seeing other family practice physicians, as well as another ENT specialist. I also saw two neurologists who referred me back to ENT. No one was able to help me. All the physicians I saw seemed baffled by my mysterious symptoms.

"Finally, in November of 1991, I was taken off the Inderal by another family practice physician who prescribed Tenormin. By this time the dizziness subsided and I went off the Antivert. From

December, 1990 till May, 1991, I was completely incapacitated and out of work — a great financial burden. Talk about stress.

"It was only recently I found information on MVPS. If only I had this years ago. I continue to take a small dose of Tenormin, and it seems to help a little. I eat a healthy diet and do aerobic exercise with strength training three to four times per week. I stopped drinking coffee and soft drinks and limited my intake of desserts. I consume a sports drink that contains natural glucose, no added sugar, and all the major electrolytes. This drink helps. My symptoms improved. I still experience extra beats and chest pain; however, now I know *why* these symptoms occur and that I *can* do something about them."

Reneé

"The term, MVP, was familiar, but the symptoms were not. In my case, MVP began with an aching, soreness, or bruising sensation in my mid-sternum area. These feelings were the first of many sensations that caused me hours of worry and concern. The original aching episode, although not severe, lasted about two days. I was able to function in my daily activities. I sought the advice of a physician who gave me my first chest X-ray in many years and my first EKG. Although both tests were negative, the sensation intermittently occurred several times a week.

"Next, I experienced shortness of breath. I didn't gasp for air, but *felt* as though I needed more air than I was able to breathe in. Again, these episodes mainly occurred when I was reading or watching TV.

"Because of these two symptoms — along with chronic fatigue, plus reoccurring headaches — I insisted something was wrong. Eventually, after two echocardiograms and a stress test, a physician diagnosed MVP. Only after I attended a lecture series on MVP did I realize that all my symptoms are fairly common. To finally know what my problem is helped decrease my stress as well as my symptoms."

Donna

"In February of 1992, after my second miscarriage, I experienced rapid heartbeats. I saw a physician, who, after an echocardiogram and an EKG diagnosed mitral valve prolapse. I began with a low dosage of Tenormin that helped some. It did not, however, help the irregular, rapid heartbeats. I avoided caffeine, alcohol, and cut down on sugar, but I felt only minimal relief.

"About a month later, I experienced extreme dizziness and lightheadedness and was treated for fluid in my ears. I was on Antivert for about one month. Shortly after, I stopped taking the Tenormin because I wanted to get pregnant again. Several tests failed to explain my two miscarriages.

"In July of 1992, I miscarried a third time. The pounding heartbeat and dizziness continued although I found some relief with routine aerobic exercise. After several infertility tests, I had surgery in October, 1992, to correct a uterine defect.

"After surgery, I continued to experience extreme dizziness, an irregular-pounding heartbeat, and a constant feeling of being off balance — like being on a boat.

"During the onset of menses when I feel stressed and tired, my symptoms magnify. I have occasional panic attacks, and I feel depressed. To always feel miserable affects both my home life and my job performance. My husband, although very understanding, often feels helpless. I am afraid to go shopping because I get dizzy and panic. I hate how it affects my life, and I hope it goes away as suddenly as it began.

"I was relieved to read *Taking Control: Living with MVPS,* and learn how other people deal with these symptoms. It helped to know panic attacks can be controlled, that positive steps can be taken. I do feel some relief from symptoms when I maintain a regular exercise schedule. Now, I am concerned about how I will be able to control my symptoms once I get pregnant, since my past history prohibits exercise."

Janet

"I am 27 years old, married and have two beautiful children. When I was five years old my pediatrician detected a heart murmur. It was not serious, and I outgrew it by the age of nine.

"Until the age of 23, my life went quite well. Then, one day when my husband and I were on our way home from Florida, I began to feel funny, tired, and dizzy. I didn't think much of it until a month later when, along with chest pains, my heart raced and palpitated. My husband rushed me to an emergency room. On the way there, I kept telling him I was scared, and I felt as if I were going to die. The physician sent me home and said there was nothing wrong with me.

"Over the next several months, my symptoms became worse. I went to several emergency rooms, and got the same response each time. 'There is nothing wrong with you — it's your nerves.'

"I experienced several anxiety, panic attacks whenever I went out. My heart raced and I felt dizzy — I had to leave. The anxiety was so intense I was scared to leave the house, and I was afraid to be alone. Eventually, I stopped driving; I stopped going any-where. I went to several physicians and specialists and asked them to help me. One said, 'It's lupus.' Another said, 'It's multiple sclerosis.' A third said, 'It's an inner-ear problem, and you need surgery.' A fourth said, 'No, you don't need surgery.' My symp-toms were very real, but the answers went from one extreme to another.

> Eventually, I stopped driving. I stopped going anywhere.

"After one year, I admitted myself into a psy-chiatric unit. Now, I had an echocardiogram. The physician told me I have MVP. I was relieved to find the cause of my symptoms, but my battle wasn't over. For the next two years, I searched for more answers to help me overcome all the fears. I saw a few other physicians who told me MVP is no big deal. It's something you have to live with.

"When I saw a newspaper ad for a class on MVP, I attended. There, I learned more about MVP in two hours than I had in two years. I joined this clinic's exercise program. When I began, every day I experienced chest pains, palpitations, migraines, fatigue, dizziness, and anxiety attacks. After six weeks of exercising three times a week and following their advice, I noticed a difference in the way I felt. I had fewer symptoms and began to feel like a new person.

"The key to reducing the symptoms and leading a normal life is to understand MVP and to know *how* to help yourself. I am fortu-nate to have a loving, supportive family."

Necia

"My problem began at a young age when the medical community seemed unaware that such a problem could exist in a child. My parents took me from physician to physician to no avail. First, I was diagnosed with anemia, given iron tablets, and told to take some type of liquid in grape juice three times a day. To spare my parents any further worry, I followed this prescription and tried to ignore my symptoms. I had nightmares, chest pain, palpita-tions, and tachycardia, as well as fatigue. If any of these prob-lems were due to a stressor, I was unaware. All I knew was at the onset I was miserable and have remained in a self-guarded state to this day.

"In school sports I was never very active — I was always the referee. I played in the symphony orchestra. As a majorette in the band, never once did I complete the parade route. I dropped out because of fatigue. Although I was an honor student and received many awards in academics and music, I did not go away to college. I was afraid to, but no one knew why.

> **I visited emergency rooms throughout the country to no avail.**

"I married a few years after my high school graduation, gave birth four years later with no problems, and remain happily married. During those years, however, I experienced numerous problems due to my condition and visited emergency rooms throughout the county to no avail. Never, until recent years, did I go to an emergency room where the staff knew what my symptoms meant. All they knew was I had a rapid, irregular heartbeat that meant trouble.

"Finally, in 1981, I was correctly diagnosed. After a scary emergency room visit and with an extremely rapid pulse that lasted for over an hour, I was admitted to the cardiac care unit and seen by a cardiologist. An angiogram — dye test of the coronary arteries — revealed that my arteries were fine. He diagnosed me with idiopathic supraventricular tachycardia — SVT, said the cause was unknown. It may come on at any time, may disappear for years and then surface at a later time. There were no instructions for my follow-up. He gave me Lanoxin and Valium, and told me to resume my life. Because I lived with this for so long with no help, I went home to live with it again.

"After taking Valium for three months and sleeping my life away, I threw the pills away and begged the physician for help. An echocardiogram revealed MVP. So now I had MVP. What a relief, but still there was no help. My primary care physician was sympathetic, but I don't believe he knew what to do.

"During my menses, my condition worsened. I would stay in bed for a week. I decided to seek help because of heavy bleeding, headache, and extreme abdominal pain. I saw a gynecologist who suggested hormone therapy. After an examination, he recommended a hysterectomy. After the hysterectomy I felt better than I had since I was a child. Ten years later I still am thankful to that gynecologist and to my primary care physician for working together to relieve me of that misery.

> **I always believed it was all in my head.**

"After the surgery, I returned to work, but the fatigue still plagued me. For several years, after work all I could do was fix dinner, maybe clean up the kitchen, and drop into bed. Then I started a walking program. Now I came home with more energy. I walked regularly for quite a while.

"Next, our son enlisted in the U.S. Marine Corps. We built a new home on the other side of the county, and I started an even more stressful job in a law office. For the next seven years I did well except for occasional tachycardia and fatigue. Then in December of 1992, while at work the tachycardia started and I could not get it under control. I went to the emergency room. Within an hour I converted on my own. I was exhausted.

"I made a follow-up appointment with a cardiologist, a wonderful, caring man. He followed my digoxin level for months and increased the dose. He also prescribed Buspar to help my panic attacks — although I did not know these were panic attacks. He instructed me to walk only for 20 minutes every other day and to not exercise any more than that. I followed his advice until late 1993.

"Because that last trip to the emergency room really scared me, I quit my job. After eight months of loneliness, I returned to work. During the time I was at home, I suffered few bouts of tachycardia.

"One day I saw an advertisement for an MVP program, called, and was sent information on a book, *Taking Control.* My prayers were answered. I read it cover to cover repeatedly, and I am grateful it was written. I have lived with this nightmare 43 years with no idea what I could do about this condition. Time and time again physicians said, 'Don't worry; it won't kill you.' I, therefore, believed it was all in my head.

"Now that I have a real handle on things, my palpitations and tachycardia don't bother me much. I no longer feel I'm in a life-threatening situation. The aftermath of exhaustion and irregular heartbeats following the tachycardia, however, take a toll on my health. Instead of hours, it now takes days to recover. I fear that as I grow older these bouts will continue to take a toll.

"I lived this nightmare by myself for 43 years. Now, it is good to know that I am correctly diagnosed, that my condition is not life threatening, and that the medical community recognizes and treats this condition. I follow advice concerning good nutrition and walk again on a regular basis. Although I still have hard beats, extra beats, and very short bouts of tachycardia, I feel rather well."

Betty

"I am now 68 years of age — healthy, active, and happy. From time to time I had a racing heartbeat and other symptoms. I wish *Taking Control* and *Network* were available when I was young. The information confirmed much of what I had learned the hard way, that is, to balance exercise and a good diet with proper rest and relaxation.

"I received two distinct benefits from reading this book. First, drink lots of fluids. Second, don't allow anyone to make me feel as though I am a hypochondriac. Thank you, especially for that."

April

"I think my symptoms started when I was nine years old. I would wake up and tell my parents I thought I was dying. My mother would stay up with me till dawn. When it began to get light outside, I felt safe enough to fall asleep. Finally, my parents scheduled a physical. The physician assured them nothing was wrong, but that I was a very emotional child. Through adolescence and into my high school years, I was constantly fearful. My fingers occasionally became numb, and I experienced shortness of breath.

> Time and time again we raced to the hospital only to be sent home.

"After age 25, my symptoms intensified. I often awakened from a sound sleep frightened and short of breath. My heart palpitated; my arms ached; and I became numb around my mouth. Although I tried to calm myself and think that it's only stress, I knew better. I continued, however, to cope on my own.

"After years of anxiety and fear, I became totally frustrated. Repeatedly, I awakened at night and asked my husband to take me to the hospital. I knew I was going to die — I was in shock. Time and time again we raced to the hospital only to be sent home. The physician assured us nothing was physically wrong. I made an appointment with a psychiatrist who prescribed sleeping pills for the night and nerve pills for the day. I wanted to know what was wrong. I asked her to put me in the hospital, run tests, and give me a complete physical examination — which she did. Still, nothing seemed wrong.

"Previous symptoms worsened. I was afraid to take the prescribed medicine because I wanted to live a normal life — to not be dependent upon medication. I tried hard to cope on my own. If I awakened, I read, did housework, or paced the floor. No one ever understood how I felt. Everyone suggested that I think more positively. Perhaps I was a hypochondriac. Try as I did, the problems remained.

"I explained to my gynecologist that I experience numbness around my mouth and a heavy feeling in my chest and arms. He admitted me to the hospital and removed a cyst from my ovary. Now that he found something wrong, I felt relieved. Perhaps I'll recover.

"During the first week following my release from the hospital, I could not sleep. For two or three weeks I averaged only two or three hours nightly. I felt as though a heavy rock rested on my chest. My arms ached. I put Bengay on them and a heating pad on my back. Nothing gave me relief.

"Again, I entered the hospital for more tests. My physician finally diagnosed MVP. At first, that scared me to death. I had a heart condition. I read books, and other literature and learned about MVP. The more I studied, the better I understood what went on inside of me for many years.

"As I go to the center to exercise and learn more about MVP, I become less fearful. It is wonderful to be involved with the MVP support group, with people who have had similar experiences. It feels good to have people finally understand me. I feel confident that with continued professional help, I will continue to conquer my fears."

Elizabeth

"As I sat in my high school physics class, I suddenly felt an odd fluttering in my chest. That's when it all started. For the next several months I made several visits to the emergency room for bouts of rapid heart rate. They said it was caffeine. On a second visit, a cardiologist suggested mitral valve prolapse and did an echocardiogram. Through my family physician, he ordered a Holter monitor. Neither physician found a sign of mitral valve prolapse.

"My family physician assured me it was just a minor arrhythmia in my heart — probably caused by stress and not dangerous. He prescribed Inderal. Because I was *not* under considerable stress, I became disturbed. I wanted to know why this happens. In fact, I hoped they really would find a prolapsed valve. Then, I would at least know what I had and that it wasn't serious.

"Fortunately, because I enjoyed dance, my cardiovascular fitness was optimal. Once I began the prescribed medication, I felt fine. Soon afterward I married and moved to Orlando. For peace of mind, I saw a cardiologist. He conducted a Doppler echocardiogram and found MVP. He never mentioned the syndrome, and I had almost no symptoms for three years.

"About six months ago, I experienced more fluttering and occasional arm pain. This started after I had gone a year without regular aerobic exercise. My job became more stressful, and I made some changes. I increased my intake of magnesium, iron, and fluids. I virtually cut out sugar and began aerobics again. I also prayed a lot. What results. I feel much better. A positive attitude helps. This syndrome is frustrating, but remember your body belongs to you — you don't belong to it. Take control."

Terry

"I am a forty-year-old female diagnosed with MVP two years ago. 'MVP is not a big deal,' said my physician. 'Live your life as normal.'

"My normal life, however, fell apart two years ago. I suffered with stress, anxiety, and panic attacks. I had more and more days of feeling bad, and I did less and less. Any exertion or any emotional change set off such symptoms as: a pounding heart, tired legs, fatigue, and lightheadedness. I lived like a robot. My family fell apart around me. They resented my feeling sick all the time. As symptoms worsened, I became disgusted, frustrated, angry, and depressed. I become agoraphobic — my fears overwhelmed me.

> **Any exertion or any emotional change set off my symptoms.**

"Then, something happened. A challenge came my way that I really wanted to meet. I knew, however, that the way I felt made it impossible to do so. I realized to feel better, I had to make changes.

"I finally found a physician who understood MVPS. He put me on medication that helped some, but not enough. Next, I attended an MVP seminar and learned so much. I wasn't going crazy; I wasn't losing my mind; and I wasn't going to die. I saw a way out of this vicious cycle that was ruling my life. I could now take charge. Out of shape, and with fears to overcome, I started a regular, low-level exercise program upon which I gradually build. I became more aware of my diet. I limited my intake of sugar and also kept fluid levels up.

"I am in a program to help me deal with agoraphobia. I aim to control my mental attitude and do not fight my symptoms and feelings. I take one day at a time. Although I have bad days, each day I take another step forward to break that vicious cycle. There is much to learn, and I am truly excited."

Arlene

"I first experienced MVP when I was 30 and pregnant with my second. I drank several cups of coffee before bedtime and couldn't sleep because of palpitations. Thereafter, I avoided caffeine and experienced no more symptoms. Three years later I was hospitalized with an irregular heartbeat for which I took two medications. It was a terrifying experience. Shortly afterward, my physician diagnosed MVP.

> **My symptoms included a fluttering feeling in my chest, and most terrifying of all, a racing heartbeat.**

"That happened nine years ago. I learned to live with my condition, in spite of trying times. My symptoms included: headaches, fatigue, palpitations, and dizziness, as well as a fluttering feeling in my chest, and — most terrifying of all — a racing heartbeat. Sometimes I feel as though I walk around in a cloud. I hate all of this.

"I started an aerobic exercise program that enabled me to go off all medication except for a half pill each day. I felt good about that. After three months, due to a couple of episodes of extremely rapid heart rate that lasted two or three minutes each, I went back on the medication.

"I now walk or ride my stationary bike daily and do well. Severe symptoms come and go during flare-ups that last several days. It's upsetting. I can't work outside my home. It's difficult to plan ahead for a nice trip. It sometimes bothers me that my problem makes things harder for my husband and sons.

"Since I receive the newsletter, *Network*, I feel hopeful knowing that many others share my problem. Now, I know there are things — both mental and physical — that we can do to feel better."

Ida

"Eleven years ago as I approached menopause, I first experienced extra heartbeats. A physician, alarmed about my extra beats, sent me to the hospital by ambulance. I was really afraid. Following tests, a cardiologist said I have MVP. My doctor told me not to worry — that it was a benign condition. My symptoms became worse — dizziness, headaches, anxiety, together with extra beats, difficult swallowing, sleep problems, ringing in my ears, and shortness of breath. I was started on Inderal and Zanax. After two years on Zanax, I became full of anxiety to the point where I couldn't go into stores. To get off Zanax, I took Ativan.

"I no longer take antidepressants, and my whole life has changed. I feel normal again, although I still have various MVP symptoms. The book *Taking Control* saved my sanity. I am no longer afraid. Recently, my physician put me on Tenormin. It didn't help much, so now I am coming off it, too. I want to see if I can take control by increasing fluids, cutting down on sugar and caffeine, and by walking. So far, this really helped me. I only wish I knew this years ago. I have had problems for ten years."

Linda

"I am a 26-year-old who was finally diagnosed with MVP two and one-half years ago. Being diagnosed was not easy. Some physicians would not listen to my symptoms. I experienced panic attacks, migraine headaches, shaking hands, unusual fatigue, and severe mood swings.

"When I could no longer keep it to myself or take another pill, I again sought help. I explained my symptoms to the physician, and that I recently graduated from college, received an offer to teach, and planned to soon marry.

"He said I was under stress and prescribed Buspar. When after a year — symptoms continued, and I was accused of suffering from PMS 365 days a year, my sister, the nurse, took over. She insisted that I be tested for MVP. My physician reluctantly complied. I had an echocardiogram, and it revealed MVP. I felt relieved because, at times, I thought I was losing my mind. Some days headaches drove me insane, and I felt like jumping out of my skin. Now, the physician prescribed Inderal.

> **I was accused of suffering from PMS 365 days a year.**

"One recent episode really frightened my husband and me. Throughout the day, I suffered palpitations, lightheadedness, and numbness in the left arm. I returned from a friend's house breathless and felt as if someone were squeezing my heart. Numbness in my left arm continued.

"At the emergency room, I had an EKG. I was told I had a prolapse episode. Again my sister began her research. She told me to call the MVP program for information. This information changed my lifestyle for the better. I cut out caffeinated products such as coffee, tea, and soft drinks. With difficulty, I cut down on chocolate.

"In retrospect, my husband remained a gem. I can't help wondering what might have happened to our marriage if I were continuously misdiagnosed. Although I still have days when I feel exhausted, it helps to be knowledgeable about MVP. I now take control of my life.

"I thank my family, my friends, my co-workers, and especially my mother — who offered prayers. You dealt with me during mood swings; you love *me* for the person I am; and I love *you.* Please wish me luck. My next venture is to get pregnant."

Phyllis

"At age 40 I still experience forceful heartbeats that began fifteen years ago. I especially notice them whenever I relax and lie on the couch.

"Because of my mother's early death that was preceded by continuing symptoms of palpitations, lightheadedness, and nausea, I shared my concern with my physician. Although he said I was too young to worry about heart trouble, he ordered an electrocardiogram. Nothing unusual showed up.

"Shortly afterward a friend said she was diagnosed with MVP. Although her symptoms resembled mine, I paid little attention. I come from a family that believes as long as you can function in your life, don't worry about it. In fact, you have to be half dead before you go to the physician. I felt pretty sure, however, that I did have MVP. Meanwhile, I learned that several years ago four of my sisters had similar symptoms. Two were on medication for palpitations and racing heartbeats.

"Two years ago I suffered from severe stress — TMJ — which my dentist eventually helped me control. A year later, I developed chest pains that recurred during stress. Sometimes, I controlled them by breathing deeply. Unfortunately, the stress and the pains continued.

> **I didn't want to do anything, to go anywhere, nor to entertain anyone.**

"I withdrew from my family and from my friends. I did not want to do anything, to go anywhere, nor to entertain anyone. All I wanted to do was sleep. Furthermore, I couldn't worry about *my* problems because my little boy began to suffer with medical problems and with scholastic problems. It got to the point where I felt exhausted all the time. My house was a mess. I became irritable, and I rejected my husband.

"After a year I felt half dead, and I became desperate. I visited another physician — explained the forceful heart beat — and he said it sounded like MVP. He said, however, my other symptoms are not usual with MVP. After blood work, chest X-ray, EKG, echocardiogram, and an upper GI test, he said my blood count was too low, and I had MVP.

"For a month I took iron pills to alleviate chest pains and fatigue. The physician believed that because the heart works harder, that might be the reason for the chest pain. To me, this made sense. After taking iron I felt better. Chest pains became less frequent, less severe. Instead of feeling exhausted by 2:30 P.M., I now remain active till at least 5:30 P.M.

"After my blood count became normal, however, the pains returned. One evening, during a very stressful week, I had a Pepsi. I couldn't get to sleep. The pains were more intense. My friend urged me to call my physician and explain the problem. I hesitated because I felt I bothered him. Although he did not believe my symptoms or physical makeup were typical of angina, he ordered a thallium stress test. The test was normal, and he prescribed Tenormin. After one week I became spaced out and almost passed out. Another time I became confused at the grocery store, unable to make decisions.

"My physician cut the medication to half a dose. He suggested that I periodically check my blood pressure. Beta blockers sometimes lower it. Although the chest pains were less severe and less frequent, I continued to feel spaced out. Next, he suggested another medication — Inderal.

"Because my husband planned a trip to San Diego and I wanted to feel good, I decided to stop the Tenormin and to not take the Inderal. I still felt tired and spaced out. As my husband and I walked the beach morning and evening, and walked afternoons to sightsee, pains became less frequent and less severe. Fatigue remained.

> I felt depressed, crazy, and began wondering if it was all in my head.

"Upon my return, I again called my physician because I felt pressure on my chest, and I was tired. He said all my tests were normal, and that he didn't tell me I *had* to take Inderal. I felt depressed, crazy, and began thinking it was all in my head. I knew it wasn't. He didn't say I was crazy, but I felt he thought I was a hypochondriac.

"A friend saw something on television about an MVP program and gave me a number to call. I did, and in turn, received valuable information. Now, I knew for sure I wasn't crazy. In fact, I was livid. Had I known about other choices other than medication, I would have chosen exercise and diet. It's a shame many professionals don't know more about MVP, don't know how to treat it, and don't know alternatives other than medication.

"I want to tell others to persist. Insist upon more tests until you find out what's wrong. Don't be intimidated as I was and assume you don't know what *you're* taking about."

Vickie

"Approximately six years ago as I stood in the middle of my living room, my heart palpitated for the first time. Prior to that I felt chest pains that lasted only a short time. Then, palpitations began on a regular basis — especially when driving. As chest pains came more frequently, I noticed several other symptoms. I had fatigue, dizziness and pain in both my arms and legs. I sought help from several physicians with no success. Finally, I visited one who gave me a complete physical. He found my electrolytes were low and I showed slight signs of hypoglycemia and low-lying asthma. He sent me to the hospital for testing. A spinal tap showed nothing. A lung test indicated slight asthma, and an echocardiogram showed MVP. He prescribed Tenormin once a day in the morning. I took the medication, and my palpitations subsided; however, I felt sick and dragged out.

"About this time I visited a cardiologist who put me on Inderal. I saw him regularly till he moved. For a few months afterward I improved. Then, my symptoms worsened. My previous physician told me to go back on Tenormin, and to take it easy. He said not to exercise too much — exercise would worsen my symptoms.

"Tenormin controlled my palpitations, but again I felt sick and dragged out. Again, I switched physicians when my medical insurance coverage changed. My new physician checked and re-checked my symptoms. I explained that my palpitations affected my ability to drive, and she suggested I see a counselor. She kept me on Tenormin and tried a calcium blocker to see if it would help. It did not.

"I met a young lady with MVP who recommended her physician because he controlled her symptoms with medication. Her doctor prescribed Lopressor and Xanax. They helped for awhile. When I tried to stop the Xanax, I felt like a lunatic. Apparently, I experienced withdrawal symptoms. I finally weaned myself and took it when my palpitations seemed they wouldn't stop. Xanax worked within 10 to 15 minutes, but it made me drowsy.

"My symptoms ranged from palpitations, anxiety, pain in my neck, numbness in my face, pain in my arms and legs, to tingling in my face and legs. Also, my nerves seemed to be shot. Frequently, whenever I drove my car, I became short of breath and experienced a swelling in the left side of my chest. Then, palpitations followed. The palpitations were severe enough that I felt helpless — as if I were dying. Sometimes I wished I would pass out to rid myself of these horrible feelings. The symptoms occurred without any pattern, and would induce an anxiety attack when I was fearful of what might occur.

"When I relax, I sometimes feel anxious, short of breath, and experience palpitations, as well as a swelling in my chest. When the symptoms become intolerable, I am frightened. I make plans with a friend and cancel because I feel bad. Friends sometimes think I'm crazy. They think all I have is a phobia about driving. I saw a psychologist who told me to drive with a friend in the car. Sometimes I feel that I do have a phobia that develops from my fear of symptoms.

> **When my symptoms are bad, I have a dreaded fear of impending death.**

"One day I read an article about people with MVP and immediately called for information. I was elated. I joined the program and exercised three times a week at the Center. I stopped my medications and noticed no difference in my symptoms. Six weeks later, I felt a difference. Anxiety and palpitations lessened, and the exercise felt great.

"Four weeks later, however, anxiety and palpitations again started every other day. Once I called 911 when I could not stop the palpitations after an hour and a half. Paramedics said both my pulse and blood pressure were up and my heartbeat was irregular. I refused to go to the emergency room because I had been there several times before to no avail. They tell you to relax. How can you when your heart is beating so rapidly? It's been six months since I discontinued my medication, and my symptoms now appear only fifty percent of the time. Once, I went an entire month without a panic attack.

"I attend an MVP support group and finally learned what causes my anxiety attacks and how to control them. Although I still have some fears and palpitations, I'm learning to deal with them. I realize panic attacks don't come out of the blue. At times I feel some anxiety about what might happen, or what angered me. When I pace myself and stop and relax between tasks, I have minimal anxiety. If, however, I allow myself to be pressured, anxiety from my symptoms turns into full-blown panic attacks. These are horrible — I avoid them at all cost."

Kathryn

"My MVP symptoms started during a trip to China — one year after retirement. Steady left-sided chest pains led to one night's stay in the emergency room. At home, two days later, a cardiologist gave me an echocardiogram that confirmed his diagnosis — MVP. 'Live a normal life; ignore the heart's pounding; and take walks. Your condition is not life threatening nor serious,' he said. He prescribed beta blockers, but I did not take them.

"Over four months, I gradually regained energy and assumed a semi-normal routine. My family physician advised me to drink more water, to use salt, and to walk. Three months later, after an appendectomy, I felt more tired. My family physician believed adrenalin surges caused my symptoms. He advised me to pace myself. My symptoms worsened. Now, I experienced chest pains, and severe nightly palpitations — severe enough that I was afraid to sleep. Twice within a week I went to the emergency room. The first time, I received a prescription for Valium and Inderal and was sent home. The second time, at my request, I was admitted and saw my cardiologist. He ordered a treadmill test and Holter monitor; both were normal.

"The cardiologist then referred me to a psychiatrist to treat my anxiety. The psychiatrist said, 'Your're running on empty,' and prescribed Xanax.

"Next, my family physician discontinued Inderal and started Tenormin. I took these medications only during potentially, stressful situations. At this time, I heard about and bought the book, *Taking Control*. After reading the book, I finally understand MVP and how to deal with it.

"Instead of Xanax, I later switched to Zoloft, that I continue to take, but in a lesser dose. Like others with MVPS, I experienced periods of not wanting to leave the house. I struggled for enough energy to function on a daily basis. With support from friends and health professionals, I improved. A health therapist convinced me I did not *have* to return to work until I am well, and when I *do* return, it should be for love — not for duty. She referred me to another therapist where, twice a month, I have acupressure and a massage. I joined relaxation classes that follow the Jon Kabit-Zinn program of stress reduction and learned how to relax — something I never knew how to do. I learned deep breathing, body scan, and sitting with awareness. Gradually, I resumed my work, and I continue to remain active. Occasionally, in times of stress, I slow down for a day or two, take a quarter of a Xanax, and — even more rarely — a Tenormin.

"I enjoy hatha yoga. It emphasizes deep, slow, breathing and meditation. Hatha yoga also complements the massage treatments and awareness training. These activities, as well as regular walking, increased my energy and diminished my symptoms. I am grateful for all the treatment, classes, and readings. I have a new understanding."

Bonnie — *a mother's point of view*

"As a mother with MVP syndrome, I find it difficult to deal with the fact my three children inherited this dominant gene. They are now young adults. However, why their lives were such a struggle was apparent only four years ago.

"We spent a great deal of time seeing physicians and enduing many medical tests. They frequently missed school. Two were even hospitalized — still without a diagnosis. My heart broke when they were told to tough it out and overcome their anxieties on their own. They were made to feel that somehow they were causing their own problems — that they were weak.

"I used to say, 'Why us? Why can't we live like a normal family?' But, today we remain much stronger and much closer than most families because we suffered together.

"I regret that I knew very little about MVPS when my children were growing up. Now, however, I *do* know and I intend to help others."

Toni and George

To conclude, let us share information about *bargaining*, a technique that encourages communication and helps people solve problems.

"MVPS affects individuals, as well as those around them — particularly family members. We, therefore, *especially* urge spouses to attend the education seminars. Their responses have been similar. For example: "I'm glad I came. Now, I understand that my wife (husband) is not the only one and isn't really crazy. She really *doesn't* make excuses. Often times, she *can't* do something or go somewhere. The seminar helped us to better understand what she is experiencing."

A true story follows. Toni, mother of six children between the ages of nine months and ten years, came with her husband — George — to the Center. Toni was sick and tired of all her symptoms. George was sick and tired of all her complaints. They both needed to find out what's wrong.

Toni was diagnosed with MVPS, and both she and George received much helpful information. A staff member recommended a home-exercise, walking program because of their geographical location and their financial difficulties. Toni became angry. Because of six children, she seldom left the house — even to go for a walk. She seldom enjoyed any free time. No doubt this pressure aggravated her symptoms. Furthermore, both said it was impossible to find anyone to watch all six children.

"Why not let George help?" said the staff member.

"Oh, no," said Toni. "I never hear the end of it when he has to watch the kids."

A discussion ensued. "She constantly complains," said George. "And, she doesn't want me to go out with my friends in the evening."

Toni thinks George doesn't understand her. George thinks Toni doesn't understand him. Obviously — anger, frustration, and bitterness prevailed. Each one complained about a lack of compassion. Because of their apparent, unsolvable problems, the staff member recommended *bargaining*.

Bargaining, a process, is a type of reciprocal behavior — something for something. For example, a couple bargains for something of equal value — something tangible, something measurable, something with a time limit.

First, each person cited a behavior that is a priority. Said Toni, "I want free time all to myself. Let George watch the kids and not complain." Toni defined free time, and George understood its meaning.

George said, "I want to go out with my friends one evening a week without Toni complaining."

They both agreed to honor their bargains for three months. One month later when asked how their bargaining was going, the response was positive. Furthermore, Toni noted a substantial decrease in her symptoms. They used bargaining with their ten-year-old son. He argues less, and he's more manageable.

As you already know, with MVPS both the symptoms and the individuals' reactions to them often present problems. Symptoms affect persons with MVPS, their families, and their friends. Symptoms may also affect working relations in a negative way. Frequent absenteeism places demands on co-workers.

Remember — there really is a light at the end of the tunnel. Learn all you can about MVPS. Share information with your family and with your friends. With a positive attitude, you will make necessary adjustments in the way you live.

References

Lederer, W. & Jackson, D. 1968. *Mirages of Marriage*. W.W. Norton & Co. New York.

Padberg, J. 1975. "Bargaining." *Perspectives in Psychiatric Care.* **13:** 68–72.

Satir, V. 1967. *Conjoint Family Therapy*. 2nd edit. Science and Behavior Books, Inc. Palo Alto, CA.

Sills, G. 1980. Nursing 806.01, "Clinical Supervision." The Ohio State University, April.

Symptom Control:
Non-drug Interventions

By yourself — without prescribed medications — decrease, and perhaps even abolish your symptoms. How?

Carefully study this chapter; then, *use* what you learn about the following.

■ **The importance of good nutrition.**

Why should I avoid caffeine?

Why should I use salt?

Why should I measure my intake of fluid?

Why concern myself with ill effects of crash diets?

Why and how should I limit my intake of sugar?

Why and how may foods possibly trigger migraines?

Why and how may a magnesium deficiency possibly affect me?

■ **The negative effects of some non-prescription drugs.**

Do some contain too much caffeine?

Do some stimulate the sympathetic system and worsen my symptoms?

■ **The positive effects of mind over matter. Move it. Exercise. Meditate.**

Why do symptoms cause me to panic, and what can I do?

Can pursed-lip breathing help to overcome shortness of breath?

Which techniques can I use to help relieve chest pains associated with MVPS?

Does stress exacerbate MVPS symptoms, and can I be helped through mindfulness meditation?

■ **The benefits derived from tangible feedback.**

Why should I monitor my progress with a *symptom checklist*?

If I study and conscientiously use non-drug intervention, may I be surprised at the end of a 12-week period?

Nutritional Aspects

Why Should I Avoid Caffeine?

Caffeine stimulates the sympathetic nervous system. It can activate, or worsen many MVPS symptoms. In fact, caffeine can produce anxiety — or panic attacks — in people with panic disorder.
Therefore, avoid caffeine altogether.

Although many foods and beverages contain caffeine, it is primarily consumed in coffee. Caffeine content of coffee, tea, cocoa
beverages, and foods varies according to the type of coffee bean,
tea leaf, or cocoa bean; method and length of brewing; and size of
serving. Caffeine content can even vary within the same brand of
coffee. For example, it's the highest in drip coffee, and the lowest
in instant coffee. Light roasted beans usually have more caffeine
than dark roasted coffee beans. (Dark beans are roasted for a
longer time, and therefore, more caffeine is burned off the bean.)
Also, contrary to popular belief, decaffeinated coffee *is not* caffeine free. Its caffeine content ranges from 2–8 mgs per 8-oz cup.

Are you hooked on caffeinated coffee? If so, start weaning
yourself now. Equallly mix caffeinated and decaffeinated coffee.
Use instant coffee — it has the lowest caffeine content. During
the next few weeks, continue to add *more* decaffeinated coffee till
you are drinking only decaffeinated coffee. If you're addicted to
caffeinated tea, follow the same procedure. Don't be alarmed if
you experience headaches. Caffeine-dependent people may temporarily suffer headaches for a week or so following withdrawal.

COMPARE CAFFEINE CONTENTS OF POPULAR FOODS AND BEVERAGE

FOOD/BEVERAGE	SERVING SIZE	CAFFEINE (mg)
Coca-Cola	12 oz can	45
Dr. Pepper	12 oz can	40
Dr. Pepper (sugar free)	12 oz can	40
Mello Yello	12 oz can	53
Mountain Dew	12 oz can	54
Mr. PiBB	12 oz can	41
Pepsi Cola	12 oz can	38
Pepsi, Diet	12 oz can	36
Royal Crown Cola	12 oz can	36
Shasta Cola	12 oz can	44
Tab	12 oz can	47

Food/Beverage	Serving Size	Caffeine (mg)
Coffee Brewed	8 oz	88
Instant	8 oz	71
Decaf	8 oz	4
Coffee — Brand Names		
Dunkin' Doughnut	10 oz	104
McDonald's	6 oz	60
Starbucks	6 oz	81
Gloria Jean's Coffee Bean	6 oz	82
The Coffee Beanery	8 oz	100
Au Bon Pain	9 oz	171
Expresso		
Starbucks	7 oz	57
Gloria Jean's Coffee Bean	2.7 oz	51
The Coffee Beanery	2.4 oz	84
Au Bon Pain	2.6 oz	130
Tea		
Brewed	6 oz	41
Instant	6 oz	29
Milk		
Chocolate	8 oz	8
Other		
Brownie, nut fudge	1-1/4 oz	8
Cake, chocolate	1/18th of 9"	14
Candy, chocolate	1 oz	8
Candy, chocolate covered	1 oz	3
Ice cream, chocolate	2/3 cup	5
Pudding, chocolate	1/2 cup	6

Source: Caffeine Labeling: Council on Scientific Affairs. *JAMA*, 252, Aug. 10, 1984; Tufts University *Diet & Nutrition Letter*, **12**: (5), July 1994.

Fluid and Salt Intake

Why Should I Use Salt?

"I have a heart problem. Shouldn't people with heart problems avoid salt?"

Although many MVPers believe this to be true, it is unwise to avoid salt, *unless*, however, you have either *high blood pressure or other medical conditions* whereby salt is restricted.

As explained in Chapter 1, MVPers may have a reduced intravascular blood volume that causes you to become lightheaded and to experience a forceful heart beat upon arising. To increase this volume, therefore, *do not* restrict salt — your source of sodium. In fact, if you aren't using salt, start now. Why?

Approximately 40% of salt is sodium, an essential mineral that retains fluid. Eat salty foods *and* drink water to help increase intravascular blood volume and decrease MVPS symtpoms. Although salt comes from natural sources such as meat and fish, most salt comes from processed foods. Examples include: soups, pickles, salsa, sauerkraut, and luncheon meats. Why should I measure my intake of fluid?

Along with maintaining your salt intake, drink a *minimum* of eight cups — two quarts — of water a day. Consume additional fluids in fruits, vegetables, juices, milk, and artificially sweetened drinks. Alcoholic and caffeinated beverages (coffee, tea, and cola) don't count. They act as diuretics and increase your body's production of urine.

To be sure to consume enough water, daily pre-measure at least 8 cups in a pitcher. Subtract the amount that you get on a regular basis from other sources. For example, if you have eight ounces of juice every morning, measure one less cup of water to your pitcher. Keep this pitcher on a kitchen counter, in the refrigerator, or on your desk at work, and take frequent drinks. For variety, add an artificially sweetened beverage mix, herbal tea, or a slice of fresh lemon or lime. Remember to fill the pitcher *daily*, and you'll know exactly how much fluid you regularly consume.

Do certain factors increase my need for water? Yes. For example, consider the atmosphere in a plane. It may have a very drying effect. Always drink plenty of fluids prior to and during the flight.[1] Be sure to ask for tomato juice — a liquid high in sodium. Too, during any illness whenever you run a fever, your body needs more water. With a fever of 103°, for example, consume at least two or three additional glasses of water daily.

During exposure to extreme heat, or during exercise when you profusely sweat, pay attention. Your thirst *may not* keep pace with your body's needs. To safely replace fluids, drink a cup of water every 20 minutes.

---

[1]MVPS is not a contraindication to flying.

Finally, avoid using diuretics or water pills. As an MVPer, you may be sensitive to these medications. On the other hand, *if* you take a prescribed diuretic, *don't stop the medication.* First, consult with your physician.

PERCENTAGES OF WATER IN COMMON FOODS	
Lettuce (iceberg)	96%
Snapbeans, radishes, celery	94%
Watermelon	93%
Cabbage (raw)	92%
Broccoli, carrots, beets, collards	91%
Orange	88%
Milk	87%
Cereals (cooked)	87%
Apples	85%
Potatoes (boiled)	80%
Bananas	76%
Eggs	74%
Corn	74%
Chicken (boiled)	71%
Fish (baked)	68%
Prunes (cooked)	66%
Beef (lean)	60%
Cheese	40%
Bread	36%
Cake (sponge)	32%
Butter	16%
Nuts	5%
Soda crackers, dry cereals	4%
Sugar (white)	trace
Oils	0%

Source: Nutritive Value of Foods, U.S. Department of Agriculture. Home and Garden Bulletin No. 72, revised 1964.

Crash or Fad Diets

Why Concern Myself with Ill Effects of a Crash Diet?

Because Americans spend millions in search of ways to lose weight, they often become vulnerable to false and sometimes adverse effects of quick-weight-loss methods: fad diets and drugs.

Fad diets are usually very low calorie diets — about 800 or less. Fad diets include: low-carbohydrate diet; high-carbohydrate diet; starvation or fasting diet; and protein-sparing modified fasts. Nutritionally inadequate diets may pose problems — particularly for MVPers who can experience changes in circulating blood volume, changes in sodium regulation, as well as changes in the autonomic nervous system.

Losses of sodium and water initially cause rapid weight loss — as much as 60% to 70%. For example, during a fasting or starvation diet, you can lose four to eight pounds within 24 hours. Also, when you initially fast, your sympathetic nervous system activity increases and sometimes increases MVPS symptoms.

Next, when you severely reduce your caloric intake, your body thinks it's starving — which it is. To compensate, your body slows its metabolism, and defeats your original purpose — to drastically reduce calories. Furthermore, your metabolism may remain low for sometime once you resume normal eating habits. Not only will you gain the weight back, you may become even heavier. Furthermore, without exercise, you lose water, fat, and muscle. You regain only fat and water. So what happens? You now replace active muscle tissue with inactive fat tissue, and slow your metabolism. Now, it becomes even *more difficult* to lose weight next time.

Something else changes: the renin-angiotensin-aldosterone system — sodium regulating mechanism. With inadequate food intake, the system may become less active and this causes sodium loss. In addition to lowering circulating blood volume, this low sodium state may lead to an increase in sympathetic nervous system activity with an increase in MVPS symptoms.

To make matters worse, some diets require diet pills. These often are thyroid or water pills. Thyroid pills can increase the actions of many bodily functions. For instance, they can cause tachycardia — increased heart rate — nervousness, irritability, and increased bowel motility. Diuretics — water pills — reduce the circulating blood volume. The ill effects of these pills, therefore, initiate or worsen MVPS symptoms.

Do know that extreme diets don't often lead to changes in food habits that support a permanent weight loss. To lose weight, you must **BURN MORE CALORIES THAN YOU CONSUME**. To safely accomplish this, moderately reduce calories, consume required nutrients, and get regular cardiovascular exercise.

Simple Carbohydrates — Sugar

Why, and how should I limit my intake of sugar?

Increased caloric intake, particularly from simple carbohydrates, sometimes increases MVPS symptoms. In fact, most calls to The MVP program about symptoms occur during the holidays. Why? Because holidays provide an excuse to indulge ourselves with pies, cakes, cookies, and candies.

When you consume sugar, especially by itself and not with a meal, there's an abrupt rise in blood glucose — blood sugar. This rise in blood glucose stimulates the secretion of insulin — the feasting hormone. Insulin stores glucose in the body's cells and lowers blood glucose. The decrease in blood glucose can stimulate epinephrine — adrenalin. The release of adrenalin can cause an increase in MVPS symptoms. It's not unusual, therefore, to hear MVPers complain of chest pains and extra beats following a mid-afternoon candy bar.

This doesn't mean that you need to totally cut sugar from your diet. Instead, fill up on nutrient-dense foods — then have an *occasional* sweet treat.

Continue to read food and beverage labels. To most people sugar is only refined white table sugar. There are, however, many sources of sugars. Any substance that ends with *ose* is a sugar. For example: Sucrose is table sugar, Lactose is milk sugar, and Fructose is fruit sugar. Sugar is also found in processed foods such as soups, spaghetti sauces, fruit drinks, cereals, and yogurts. Too, sugar occurs naturally in fruits, vegetables, and dairy products.

Always study the ingredient list. Items are listed by weight in *descending order* according to their content. Therefore, be careful if sugar is listed first. This product contains a higher content of sugar than one in which sugar is listed *at the end* of the label. Beware that many manufactures call sugar by several different names. The amount of sugar in a product is sometimes misleading. For example, a granola cereal may have rolled oats listed first, brown sugar second, corn syrup third, and honey fifth. Since *all* of these are sugars, sugar makes up most of this product.

Avoid concentrated sugars — not fructose and lactose. Resist the temptation to snack on candy bars, pastries, and doughnuts — especially by themselves. If you crave M & M's or a Reese's cup — first eat a well-balanced meal. Then eat a sugary treat. Why? Nutrients such as fat, protein, and complex carbohydrates take longer to digest than sugar does. Therefore, your blood sugar may remain more stable than if you ate a concentrated, sugary food by itself.

Reduce sugar in baking. Examples: Sugar usually can be reduced by 1/3 and it won't affect the recipe. To add flavor, experiment with spices such as: cinnamon, cardamon, coriander, nutmeg, ginger, and mace. Avoid soft drinks or sodas. Prefer water with a piece of lemon or lime. Choose fruit for dessert. Fruit has a high water content and few calories. Use fructose instead of sucrose — table sugar. Fructose is 70% sweeter than sucrose, and you don't need as much.

TEASPOONS OF SUGAR IN COMMON FOODS

FOOD	SERVING SIZE	TEASPOONS SUGAR
Chewing gum	1 stick	1/2
Gingersnaps	1 medium	1
Marshmallow	1 average	1-1/2
Jam	1 tablespoon	3
Honey	1 tablespoon	3
Hamburger bun	1 bun	3
Caramel	3 pieces	4
Lowfat yogurt, plain	1 cup	4
Tang	8 ounces	4
Fruit cocktail	1/2 cup	5
Angel food cake	1/12 cake	6
Kool-Aid	8 ounces	6
Sherbet	1/2 cup	6–8
Soft drink	12 ounces	6–9
Apple pie	1/6 medium pie	12
Lowfat yogurt, fruited	1 cup	13
Chocolate cake, iced	1/12 cake	15

Sources: Brody, J. 1987. "Jane Brody's Nutrition Book." Bantam Books. New York. Pennington, J., & Church, H. 1989. "Food Values of Portions Commonly Used." (15th edit.). J.B. Lippincott Co. Philadelphia.

Satisfying that Sweet Tooth

Do you have a sweet tooth? Can't live without that chocolate bar? Then, try these sweet recipes. They use little or no sugar, and are lower in saturated fat. For other recipes, see the references listed at the end of this chapter.

Flavorful Yogurt
INGREDIENTS:
> 8 ounces plain nonfat or lowfat yogurt
> 1 capful of vanilla or almond extract
> sweetener to taste — such as 2–3 packets of Nutrasweet
> 1/4 cup fresh chopped fruit (optional) such as strawberries
>   or peaches

DIRECTIONS: Mix all ingredients together. Refrigerate or freeze. Great as a snack or dessert. Serves 1.

*Granola Apple Crisp**
INGREDIENTS:
> 6 medium apples, peeled, cored, and sliced
> 1 tablespoon whole wheat flour
> 3/4 teaspoon cinnamon
> 1/4 teaspoon ground nutmeg
> 3/4 cup apple juice
> 1/4 cup packed brown sugar
> 3 tablespoons whole wheat flour
> 1/4 teaspoon cinnamon
> 1/4 teaspoon salt
> 1/4 cup margarine
> 1/2 cup quick or old-fashioned oats
> 3 tablespoons bran-type cereal or wheat germ
> 3 tablespoons chopped walnuts or pecans
> 1 teaspoon toasted sesame seeds

DIRECTIONS: In a bowl, stir together apples, 1 tablespoon flour, 3/4 teaspoon cinnamon, and 1/4 teaspoon nutmeg. Turn into an 8 x 8 x 2 baking dish. Build up edges slightly. Pour apple juice over fruit.

In another bowl, combine brown sugar, remaining flour, 1 teaspoon each of cinnamon and salt. Cut in margarine until well blended. Stir in remaining ingredients and sprinkle over fruit in center. Leave a ring of apples showing around edge.

Bake at 375 degrees for 30 minutes. Serves 8.

*Reprinted with permission from the greater Cincinnati Nutrition Council's Cookbook, *Nutritious and Delicious*, 1985.

Simple Apple Treat
INGREDIENTS:
    1 apple cored, peeled, and sliced
    cinnamon to taste (about 1/8 teaspoon)
    dash of nutmeg (optional)
    sweetener (optional)
DIRECTIONS: Place sliced apples on a microwave-safe plate. Sprinkle cinnamon and a dash of nutmeg on top (optional). Cook in the microwave 3–5 minutes on high power till the desired consistency. Add sweetener such as Nutrasweet (optional). Serves 1.

Baked Banana
Place a whole ripe *unpeeled* banana on a cookie sheet. Bake at 350° for 20 minutes. Split the banana a with knife; sprinkle with cinnamon or nutmeg.

Raspberry Cheesecake
INGREDIENTS:
    Pre-made graham cracker crust
    1 package sugar-free raspberry flavored gelatin
    1 cup boiling water
    1 container (16 ounces) lowfat cottage cheese
    1 cup part skim ricotta cheese
    2 cups fresh raspberries
DIRECTIONS: Stir sugar-free raspberry gelatin and boiling water until completely dissolved. Set aside until lukewarm. In a blender or food processor, blend cottage and ricotta cheeses until smooth; pour into large bowl. Blend in reserved gelatin mixture. Pour filling into crust. Chill until almost firm (about 3 hours). Top with 2 cups of raspberries. Chill at least 2 more hours. Serves 12.

Sugarless Cookies
INGREDIENTS:
    1-3/4 cups flour
    2 teaspoons baking powder
    1/2 teaspoon salt
    1/2 teaspoon cinnamon
    3/4 cup orange juice
    1/2 teaspoon grated orange rind
    1/2 cup minus 1 tablespoon vegetable oil
    1 egg
    1/2 cup chopped walnuts
    1/2 cup raisins

DIRECTIONS: Preheat oven to 375° F. Combine dry ingredients. Add remaining ingredients; mix well. Drop by teaspoon on ungreased cooking sheet to make 32-34 cookies. Bake about 15 to 20 minutes. When done, remove from pan and cool.

VARIATIONS:

Add 1/4 teaspoon ground cloves for a spice drop.

Instead of raisins, add 1/2 cup chopped or whole cranberries.

Source: *Family Cookbook*. Volume I. 1987. The American Diabetes Association and The American Dietetic Association.

Foods and Migraines

Why and How May Foods Possible Trigger Migraines?

Migraines can be triggered by food, as well as by a combination of other factors. It's believed that natural and artificial biochemicals contained within foods trigger headaches. For example, some migraine sufferers are deficient in the enzyme that digests amines. Therefore, any foods that contain the amino acid tyramine — or other amines — may cause migraines.

It's believed that tyramine acts either directly, or indirectly, through the release of norepinephrine — a powerful vasoconstrictor. Norepinephrine affects sensitive blood vessels that can cause a migraine attack. You'll find tyramine in foods and beverages such as cheddar and bleu cheese, and red wines that undergo bacterial decomposition.

Also, migraines can be triggered by eating foods containing nitrites such as: hot dogs, bacon, sausage, and ham — cured meats. Additives, such as monosodium glutamate — MSG — found in some TV dinners and in some foods from Chinese restaurants, can also trigger migraines. Many others, who suffer with migraines, however, must learn to recognize and avoid foods to which they are sensitive.

As a precautionary measure, avoid foods containing amines. Instead of aged cheeses such as Swiss, cheddar, or provolone, choose Ricotta, cottage, or American cheese. If red wine, brandy or beer trigger a migraine, drink white wine. Choose freshly prepared meat rather than canned or aged ham, bacon, sausage, hot dogs, or dried fish. If yeast breads — white, or sourdough breads — trigger an attack, eat whole wheat and rye breads.

Herbs that can be effective in the treatment of migraine headaches include: feverfew, ginkgo biloba extract, peppermint, rosemary, and wormwood. Feverfew helps alleviate pain and ginkgo biloba enhances cerebral circulation.

Keep a food diary. Then, see what you ate *prior* to each migraine attack. Try to identify the culprits. Avoid them for a trial period of time, and see what happens.

Magnesium Intake

Why and How may a Magnesium Deficiency Possibly Affect Me?

As mentioned in Chapter 1, there's evidence that magnesium deficiency may play a role in MVPS symptoms. Therefore, avoid diets high in fats. Fat substances inhibit the absorption of magnesium. Dietary phosphates — very high in certain sodas — also inhibit reabsorption of magnesium. Study the following chart, and limit your intake of soft drinks high in phosphates.

PHOSPHATE CONTENT IN SOFT DRINKS

SOFT DRINK	PHOSPHORUS (mg)
Dr. Pepper	44
Diet Dr. Pepper	44
Caffeine-free Dr. Pepper	44
Coca-Cola classic	41
Caffeine-free Coca-Cola classic	41
Coke II	38
Cherry Coca-Cola	37
TAB	30
Diet Mr. PiBB	29
Mr. PiBB	29
Diet Coke	18
Caffeine-free diet Coke	18
Diet cherry Coca-Cola	18
PowerAde fruit punch	2
PowerAde orange	2
Welch's sparkling grape soda	34
Sprite	0

Soft Drink	Phosphorus (mg)
Diet Sprite	0
Minute Maid orange	0
Diet Minute Maid orange	0
Mello Yello	trace
diet Mello Yello	trace
Fresca	trace
Fanta orange	0
7Up	only as present in water
Diet 7Up	only as present in water

Source: Consumer Information Center, The Coca-Cola Company 1/94; Consumer affairs, Dr. Pepper/Seven-Up Corporation 4/94.

Refining foods, especially white sugar and grains, causes large losses of magnesium. In cooking and baking, substitute brown sugar for white. One-half cup of brown sugar contains 20 milligrams of magnesium; white sugar has none. Steam — don't boil vegetables — to preserve magnesium.

MVPers should get an adequate amount of magnesium daily — 350 mg for men, 280 mg for women — by eating a well-balanced diet. Good sources of magnesium include: nuts, legumes, cereal grains, green leafy vegetables, apples, apricots, avocados, bananas, blackstrap molasses, brewer's yeast, brown rice, figs, garlic, kelp, lima beans, peaches, wheat, and whole grains.

As MVPers, exercise caution, and *never assume that you're deficient in magnesium. Don't take upplements without first consulting your physician.* Magnesium supplements may be unnecessary, or even forbidden, as for example, with impaired renal — kidney function.

On the other hand, provided magnesium supplements *are* advised, consider the following facts. Some multivitamin pills contain magnesium oxide and are poorly absorbed. Likewise, some contain magnesium salts — magnesium hydroxide — used as laxatives and are also poorly absorbed. Too, oral magnesium supplements sometimes cause gastrointestinal side effects such as nausea and diarrhea.

Magnesium supplements with high solubility in sustained-release forms offer the best tolerability and bioavailability. (Bioavailability refers to the degree of a drug's availability to the body's tissues after administration.) If your physician recommends oral-magnesium therapy, dosage may range from 400-600 mg.

Non-prescription Drugs

The Negative Effects of Some Non-prescription Drugs

Do some contain too much caffeine?

There are a number of non-prescription drugs, or over-the-counter — OTC — medications that contain caffeine. Some of these include Anacin, Excedrin Extra-Strength, Midol, Nodoz, Vanquish, and Vivarin. Read labels. Avoid medications that contain adrenalin, adrenalin-like substances, and caffeine.

CAFFEINE CONTENT OF NON-PRESCRIPTION DRUGS

NON-PRESCRIPTION DRUG	MG/TABLET OR CAPSULE
Anacin Analgesic	32
Cope	32
Dexatrim	200
Dristan	32
Excedrin	65
Midol	32
Nodoz	100
Neo-synephrine	15
Prolamine	140
Sinarest	30
Triaminicin	30
Vanquish	33
Vivarin tablets	200

Source: Pennington, J., & Church, H. "Food Values Of Portions Commonly Used." 1985, 14th edit., Harper & Row Publishers. New York.

Do some contain other stimulants that may worsen my symptoms?

There are many non-prescription drugs that contain ephedrine and pseudoephedrine. Ephedrine and pseudoephedrine stimulate the sympathetic system and may worsen MVPS symptoms. Examples include: Actifed, Benadryl, Chlor-Trimeton, Drixoral Antihistamine, Congestac, CoTylenol, Novahistine DMX, Robitussin-PE, Sinutab, Sine-Aid, Tylenol Maximum Strength and Sudafed. (For information on antihistamines and decongestants, see Chapter 8.)

The Positive Effects of Mind Over Matter. Move It. Exercise. Meditate

Move It

Can you identify with this scenario? As you sit and watch TV, or as you sit at a desk, you suddenly feel a flip-flop sensation from those nasty extra beats. "I'm having a heart attack. I *know* this time it's fatal," you say to yourself.

What do you do? You take your pulse. One skipped beat, two skipped beats, three skipped beats. "Oh no, this IS it."

And what do you keep doing? You continue to sit, and you continue to take your pulse. Your sense of fear intensifies and makes matters worse. You become even more frightened. Your nervous system releases more and more adrenalin. Now, the chest pains begin. What can I do?

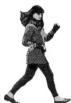 Don't sit. Don't panic. Don't take your pulse. Instead, *move it.* Get up; get busy; or take a walk. As you do, your heart rate increases and usually overrides — or suppresses extra beats. Furthermore, when you're busy you refocus your energies *on the task and not on the extra heartbeats*.

Janet, one of our program participants who formerly sat, checked her pulse, and panicked when she experienced extra beats, followed our advice. Now, every time she feels extra beats, she vacuums.

"This idea works," she said, "and I also have the cleanest house in town."

Pursed-lip Breathing

Can pursed-lip breathing help to overcome shortness of breath?

Pursed-lip breathing effectively helps many MVPers overcome their inability to take a deep breath. Therefore, whenever you feel breathless, take a breath — any kind — through your nose. Next, *slowly* breathe out through your mouth with your lips pursed — as if you're blowing out a candle. Don't breathe out through your nose.

Again, take a breath — a deeper one. To exhale, repeat. Breathe out *slowly* through pursed lips. Repeat the cycle till you can take full, deep breaths. Remember to always *breathe out slowly* through pursed lips, and after three or four breaths, you should feel relief.

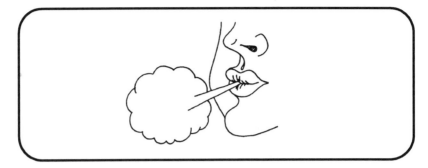

Feet Up

Which techniques can I use to help relieve chest pains associated with MVPS?

Lie down on your back and bend your knees, or raise your legs. Place your legs either on a couch or against the wall. The chest pain often subsides within a few minutes.

Of course, this isn't always feasible, particularly if you're at work or in a crowded shopping mall. Here's a variation. Sit crossed-legged (Indian style), and lean your head forward toward your knees.

Do know, these techniques *are not* appropriate treatments for chest pains caused by other medical conditions.

Exercise

Because exercise is a *key factor* in reducing the frequency, intensity, and severity of MVPS symptoms, it is discussed in detail in the next chapter.

Stress and Mindfulness Meditation

Does stress exacerbate MVPS symptoms, and can I be helped through mindfulness meditation?

Daily living causes both outer and inner stressors. Typical outer stressors result from people stress, time stress, and role stress. Inner stressors, on the other hand, relate to physical, mental, and emotional states such as fatigue, obsessive thinking, and anxiety or depression.

If stressors cause a significant stress reaction and increase activity of the autonomic nervous system — ANS — *yes*, they may activate or even worsen MVPS symptoms. And, no drugs by themselves provide immunity to stress or pain and solve life's problems.

Each one of us must realize the futility of expecting *someone else* to make things better. Although some forces are beyond our control, others really are not. To a great extent, *we* influence circumstances by the way we see things. How we see things determines how much energy we have and how we positively channel that energy in the right direction. Such energy comes from inside, is within our reach, and is within our potential control. How can we tap into it? Cultivate mindfulness meditation and discover deep realms of relaxation, calmness, and insight.

What, then, is mindfulness meditation? Mindfulness is an ancient practice of being in the present moment fully and feeling each moment as a new beginning. It is a way of paying attention, a way of looking deeply within oneself to gain understanding. There is a way to look at problems, to come to terms with problems, and to make life more joyful *when you are in control*. This is a way of being, a way of awareness, a way of mindfulness. Unlike familiar forms of meditation that involve focusing on a sound, a phrase, or a prayer to minimize distracting thoughts, mindfulness recommends the opposite. Rather than ignore distracting thoughts, sensations, or physical discomfort — focus on them.

As an MVPer, challenge your mindfulness. Say to yourself, "Right now I live my life, and I make many choices. In a stressful situation, I *choose* to react; or I *choose* to calmly respond."

Therefore, whenever you're stressed, don't feel helpless or adopt a fight-or-flight solution. Instead, let mindfulness — moment-to-moment awareness help you to take control. Increase your level of awareness and decide *how* to manage it for the better.

To do so, bring your awareness to your face and shoulders as they tense up, to your heart as it pounds, to your lungs if you're breathless, or to any other needy part of your body. Again, say to yourself, "I *choose* to overcome it."

Next, focus on your breath. Your breath reconnects you with calmness, and brings you to an awareness of your whole body. To meditate, *feel* the movement of air as it flows in and out past your nostrils. *Feel* the movement of your chest as it expands and contracts. Don't push or force each breath. Simply *be aware* of its feeling. As you do so, with each breath you center not on the past nor in the future. You center on the *present* moment. Your mind and your body unite in the present.

NOTE: Although you learn to respond to stress with awareness, it doesn't mean you'll never react or become overwhelmed by anger, grief, or fear. Instead, you'll gradually learn how to control and how to deal with stress. The idea isn't to suppress your emotions, but to learn how to control and deal with them. To respond to stress requires moment-to-moment awareness. Take each moment as it comes.

Body-scan Meditation

Following a hectic day, use the body scan before retiring. Lie on your back and focus your mind throughout different regions of your body. Begin with the toes of one foot, up the leg to the pelvis and feel the sensations as you direct your breath to and from each region. Repeat the procedures on the other foot and leg. Next, direct your breath to remaining parts of your body till you reach the top of your head. End up by breathing through an imaginary hole in the top of your head. Throughout the scan as you imagine the placement of each breath, also imagine feelings of fatigue and tension as they flow out each time you exhale. Believe that each *new* breath brings vitality and relaxation.

Sitting Meditation

Sit in a comfortable position and focus on your breath. Soon your attention wanders to various thoughts, feelings, or body sensations. With this practice you note thoughts, feelings and body sensations; but, you don't dwell on them. Instead, you direct your attention to your breathing. Use sitting meditation upon arising to clear your mind, center your thoughts, and give you renewed clarity and energy.

Walking Meditation

Enjoy a walk with nowhere to go, no time to be there. Fully experience your body as you walk on earth during this time frame. Take purposeful steps, placing your heel, then toes on the ground. Feel the earth beneath you.

Mindful Hatha Yoga

Another technique helpful in lessening MVPS symptoms is mindful hatha yoga — gentle stretching and strengthing exercises, with moment-to-moment awareness of breathing and bodily sensations during various postures. As one program participant says, "Through yoga, I learned how to relax, and how to breathe. I learned that you can't relax till you're breathing correctly. It takes time to learn, but the time is well spent. I also know that not every bodily sensation is MVPS related. Now, I can deal with these sensations — and not panic. Before learning yoga, I did. Yoga helped me effectively deal with my MVPS symptoms, and I'm more at peace with myself."

A complete description of mindfulness training is beyond the scope of this chapter. If interested in learning more about these practices, see references listed at the end of the chapter. In addition, check your local newspaper for meditation programs.

Tangible Feedback

The Benefits Derived from Tangible Feedback

Why should I monitor my progress with a symptom check list?

Now that you're aware of interventions that help to control MVPS symptoms, monitor your progress with the *symptom check list*. It was originally developed for a research study. The check list was used to monitor symptoms of MVPS on a weekly basis, and to note changes over time. Since its development, many MVPers used the symptom check list to assess their progress. It's one way to note your improvements.

Take a moment now and complete the check list. Think of the past week. Which symptoms did you experience, and how frequent were they? If you experienced chest pain every day, place a five in the frequency column opposite chest pain. If you had palpitations or extra beats one or two times for the entire week, then place a one next to this symptom.

Start using the non-drug interventions you've learned. At the end of each week, fill out this check list. Do so for twelve weeks. You'll be pleased at how well you do.

Next, take a piece of graph paper and plot the frequency numbers for each symptom over 12 weeks. On the left-hand side of the graph write the numbers 0 to 5 — or 0 to 3 if you never had higher than a 3. On the bottom, write the weeks 1 to 12. What you'll see is an overall decrease in the frequency of your symptoms.

The following example is from a research study done at the MVPPC. The weekly average of the frequency for the symptom mood swings for the exercise group and the control group — nonexercise group — are plotted over 12 weeks. Note the difference between the two groups, and the decrease in frequency of mood swings in the exercise group.

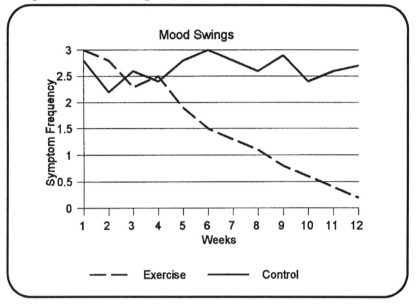

MOOD SWINGS

Another idea is a behavioral chart developed by an MVPer. Use this chart in combination with the symptom check list.

BEHAVIOR	POOR	FAIR	GOOD	EXCELLENT
Sugar intake				
Water intake				
Sodium intake				
Exercise				
Stress				
Personal schedule				

Submitted by: M. Goodwin, Belleville, Illinois. 1992.

If you're eating lots of chocolate or other sweets, then check *poor* for sugar and caffeine intake. In other words, you did a poor job of following advice for symptom control. If you feel under lots of stress, then check *poor* next to stress. If you overbooked yourself — many places to go and not enough time — check *poor* next to personal schedule.

SYMPTOM CHECK LIST

Name_____Week # ____ Week ending ___/___/___

Please place a number next to the symptom that best indicates the frequency with which you experienced this symptom during the **past week**:

5 - All of the time
4 - Most of the time
3 - A good bit of the time
2 - Some of the time
1 - A little of the time
0 - None of the time

SYMPTOM	FREQUENCY
Chest pain and/or chest discomfort	
Arm pain and/or arm discomfort	
Palpitations/extra beats/Skipped beats/heart pounding	
Shortness of breath	
Fatigue	
Headache	
Anxious (feeling nervous or frightened)	
Mood swings	
Dizziness and/or lightheadedness	
Passing out spells (losing consciousness)	
Muscle cramps	

I saw my physician ___Yes ___No. If yes, was this a routine visit? ___ Yes___No.

I missed ___days from work.

I went to the emergency room for treatment. ___Yes ___No.

Copyright © K.A. Scordo, 1988. All rights reserved. Reproduction in whole or part by any means whatsoever without written permission is prohibited.

Selected References

Balch, J., & Balch, P. 1990. *Prescription for Nutritional Healing.* Avery Publishing Group, Inc. Garden City Park, New York

"Brewed Coffee." October, 1994. *Consumer Reports.* **69:** 640–651.

Feuerstein, G. & Bodian, S. (Eds.) 1993. *Living Yoga: A Comprehensive Guide for Daily Life.* Putnam Publishing Group. New York.

Gaffney, F., & Blomqvist, C. 1988. "Mitral valve prolapse and autonomic nervous system dysfunction: A pathophysiological link." In: *Mitral Valve Prolapse and the Mitral Valve Prolapse Syndrome* (H. Boudoulas & C. Wooley, Eds.). Futura Publishing Co., Inc. New York. 427–443.

Galland, L., Baker, S., & McLellan, R. 1986. "Magnesium deficiency in the pathogenesis of mitral valve prolapse." *Magnesium* **5**: 165–174.

Harris, S. 1995. "White Light Yoga" (Video). For additional information, Sara Harris, 4 City Hall Road, Accord, New York 12404.

Kabat-Zinn, J. 1990. *Full Catastrophe Living: Using the Wisdom of Your Body and Mind to Face Stress, Pain, and Illness.* Delta. New York.

Kabat-Zinn, J., Massion, A., Kristeller, J. *et al.* 1992. "Effectiveness of a meditation-based stress-reduction program in the treatment of anxiety disorders." *American Journal of Psychiatry*, 936–943.

Klein, M. 1994. "Magnesium therapy in cardiovascular disease." *Cardiovascular Review and Report.* 9-27.

Pennington, J., & Church, H. 1985. *Food Values of Portions Commonly Used.* 14th edit. Harper & Row Publishers. New York.

Scordo, K. 1991. "Effects of aerobic exercise training on symptomatic women with mitral valve prolapse." *American Journal of Cardiology.* **67:** 863–867.

Solomon, S. 1991. *The Headache Book.* Consumer Reports Books.

Toseland, R. & Rivas, R.1984. *An Introduction to Group Work Practice.* MacMillian Publishing Co. New York.

Watkins, P., & Russell, R. 1990. "Mitral Valve Prolapse Syndrome 1990: Appropriate diagnosis is key to a happy patient." *Illustrated Medicine.* **5:** 1–15.

Exercise and MVPS

"Exercise? I can hardly get out of bed in the morning."
"I have to conserve my limited energy."
"I have no time — I'm too busy."
"I'm afraid to exercise. Something terrible will happen."

Sound familiar? Some MVPers fear the consequences of exercise. Others fear a need to conserve limited energy. Do know inactivity causes deconditioning — an undoing of physical fitness. *Symptoms do not decrease with inactivity — they increase.*

Deconditioned people experience reduced-exercise tolerance — they can't do as much, or last as long. Deconditioning causes symptoms similar to those of MVPS. It often becomes difficult to determine where deconditioning symptoms end, and where deconditioning symptoms of MVPS begin. For instance, as with MVPers, deconditioned people have high resting heart rates. This is analogous to racing a car's engine when it's idling. Then, with minimal activity, there is a rapid, inappropriate increase in heart rate. This causes shortness of breath, and feelings of fatigue that lead to further inactivity. Thus, the cycle continues. The less you do, the less you feel like doing. This cycle, however, can be broken with regular cardiovascular exercise.

Although regular cardiovascular exercise benefits many people, it particularly benefits MVPers (see list on next page). Those who regularly exercise have less symptoms and more endurance than those who don't.

Physical fitness not only helps you get the most out of life, it also helps equip you to meet everyday demands. Regardless of either your age or your present level of fitness, you'll benefit from a program of proper cardiovascular exercise.

**IMPORTANT CARDIOVASCULAR TRAINING EFFECTS:
BENEFITS FOR MVPERS**

- Lowered plasma catecholamines — epinephrine or adrenalin and norepinephrine — believed responsible for some mvps symptoms

- Lowered resting heart rate

- Increased maximal cardiac output — the amount of blood the heart pumps in one minute at peak exercise

- Decrease in heart rate at any matched submaximal work load — lower heart rate while doing the same amount of work

- Increase in both maximal and submaximal stroke volume — the amount of blood pumped out of the heart ventricles with each beat

- Increase in resting-blood volume

- Improvement of stress management, reduction of the effects of stress, and a quicker recovery from psychosocial stress

- Increased alertness and self-confidence

- Increased endurance and energy level

- Promotion of a sense of well-being

What is Physical Fitness?

The President's Council on Physical Fitness and Sports defined physical fitness as "the ability to carry out daily tasks with vigor and alertness, without much fatigue, and with enough energy to enjoy leisure-time pursuits, and to meet unforeseen emergencies." In other words, you should have not only enough energy to survive, but enough energy to enjoy life.

> **COMPONENTS OF PHYSICAL FITNESS**
>
> • Cardiorespiratory fitness
>
> • Flexibility
>
> • Muscular fitness
>
> • Body composition

The four components of physical fitness include:

(1) Cardiorespiratory — aerobic — fitness: the ability of the heart, lung, and circulatory system to take in, deliver, and use oxygen needed for cellular-energy production. Aerobic fitness enhances endurance and lessens MVPS symptoms. (You may measure your level of cardiorespiratory fitness by a graded exercise stress test.)

(2) Flexibility: the maximum ability to move a joint through a range of motion. For example, the trunk flexion or sit-and-reach test evaluates hamstring and low-back flexibility. Adequate flexibility is important for activities that require bending and stretching. Flexibility is also important for preventing injury and soreness during activities. MVPers often have increased joint flexibility.

(3) Muscular fitness — two types of muscular fitness: The first is muscular strength — the maximal force generated by a specific muscle or muscle group. For example, the heaviest weight you lift one time on a leg extension is the muscular strength of your quadriceps — the group of muscles in the front of your thigh. Activities such as carrying groceries or carrying small children require varying degrees of muscular strength.

The second type of muscular fitness is muscular endurance — the ability of a muscle group to exert a less-than-maximal force for an extended period of time. Exercises such as biking and rowing require muscular endurance.

(4) Body Composition: the percentage of your weight that is fat — % body fat. Body composition is more important than actual weight. For example, your weight might be within the proper range on a height-and-weight chart, but your percentage

of body fat is high. Conversely, you might be overweight on the chart, but in actuality be slender and have good muscle tone. To calculate an ideal body weight, therefore, consider your body composition. Don't rely on only a height-and-weight chart.

Together, these components constitute overall physical fitness. Not every exercise, however, improves *all* of these components. For example, although doing house work, carrying groceries, and lifting weights are work, they are not considered cardiovascular exercise. Therefore, these activities lack the important symptom-controlling benefits of regular aerobic exercise.

Types of Exercise and Their Benefits

Aerobic Exercise

Aerobic means with oxygen. Aerobic — endurance — exercise uses oxygen to produce energy. Moderate in intensity, aerobic exercise involves the rhythmic movement of large muscle groups. This type of exercise conditions the cardiovascular system. Examples include: bicycling, jogging, rowing, swimming, brisk walking, and cross-country skiing. Aerobic exercise also improves muscular endurance and body composition — two components of fitness. Fat is burned, muscle tone is increased, and body composition is improved.

Short Term — Acute — Effects of Aerobic Exercise

Acute effects of exercise include: an increase in heart rate, stroke volume — the amount of blood the heart pumps each beat, and cardiac output — the amount of blood the heart pumps in a minute. These effects help meet the increased demand for oxygenated blood, and create additional energy required for exercise. Aerobically untrained MVPers, however, tend to have greater heart-rate increases than those aerobically untrained people *without* MVPS.

Exercise also effects blood pressure. Systolic blood pressure — upper number in a blood pressure reading — is the pressure in arteries when the heart contracts. Diastolic blood pressure — the lower number in a blood pressure reading — is the pressure in arteries between heart beats. Normally to meet the increased demand for blood, systolic pressure increases with activity and diastolic pressure remains the same.

Exercise also decreases circulating-stress hormones — adrenalin and its related substances. Following exercise, you feel relaxed and more alert.

Training Effects of Aerobic Exercise

Training effects — long-term benefits — of regular aerobic exercise begin within six to eight weeks. By then, most MVPers notice a decrease in symptoms.

With cardiovascular training, your resting heart rate becomes lower and your heart rate's response to exercise improves. Now, when you climb a flight of stairs, your heart rate increases to only 90 beats per minute, instead of 150 beats as it did three months ago. In essence, you taught your cardiovascular system how to function more economically.

Intravascular blood volume and cardiac output increase with cardiovascular training. This helps alleviate the forceful heart beat and any feeling of lightheadedness when you stand up. Furthermore, blood levels of the adrenalin-like substances — catecholamines — may decrease. This may lessen the extra beats, chest pains, anxiety and other MVPS symptoms.

Training effects also improve muscle tone, muscular endurance, and your body's response to other activities. But, these cardiovascular training effects last *only* if you continue regular exercise. Once you stop, you can lose the benefits of aerobic conditioning within two weeks. To receive continued benefits, therefore, plan to exercise throughout your lifetime.

Anaerobic

Anaerobic exercise, such as sprinting or strength training, is high-intensity exercise that uses glycogen — carbohydrates stored in the muscles. This type of exercise causes a rapid depletion of glycogen stores and the build-up of lactic acid. Although anaerobic exercise doesn't benefit the cardiovascular system, it does increase muscular strength — a component of fitness.

Types of Muscular Strength Training

(1) Isotonic — same tension: Isotonic contractions occur when a weight is held constant while the muscle shortens and lengthens. Examples of isotonic exercise include: pushups,

situps, lifting free weights and using weight stations such as Universal machines.

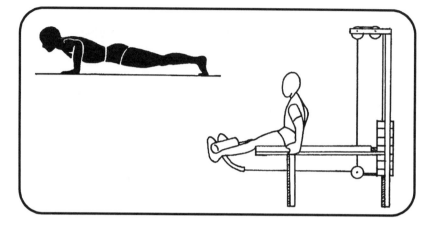

EXAMPLES OF ISOTONIC CONTRACTIONS

(2) Isokinetic — same movement: Isokinetic contractions occur as a muscle shortens to counteract aresistance developed by a special machine. The speed of the contraction remains constant and the resistance to the contraction remains proportional to the force exerted. In other words, the harder you push or pull, the more resistance you feel while the speed remains the same. You accomplish isokinetic muscle contractions with expensive mechanical equipment such as a Cybex dynamometer (Lumex, Bayshore, NY). Competitive athletes use this equipment to improve their range of joint motion. Others use isokinetic exercise to rehabilitate injured muscles. For most people, however, isokinetic exercise equipment is unnecessary.

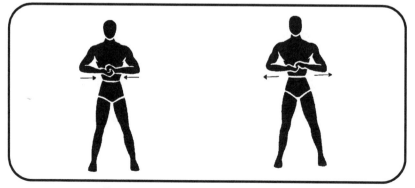

EXAMPLE OF ISOMETRIC CONTRACTIONS

(3) Isometric — same measure: Isometric — static — muscular contractions occur when muscular tension develops without much muscle movement. An example of an isometric contraction is pushing your hands together to create tension without moving your arms. Other examples include carrying heavy luggage, or carrying heavy bags of groceries. Isometric contractions can cause abrupt rises in blood pressure. Therefore, people with hypertension — high blood pressure — should avoid this type of strength training. Because of abrupt blood volume changes, isometric exercises should generally be avoided by MVPers.

> *The most important type of exercise for people with MVPS is aerobic exercise. This form of exercise produces the physiological adaptations that reduce the frequency and intensity of MVPS symptoms.*

The Exercise Prescription: Aerobic Exercise

Each exercise prescription is designed to enhance physical fitness, promote health, and ensure one's safety during participation. Exercise prescriptions vary with a person's interests, needs, background, and health status. The most desirable exercise prescription, however, helps you to habitually increase your physical activity and to decrease your MVPS symptoms. A discussion of the five components of an exercise prescription — intensity, mode, duration, frequency, and progression of physical activity — follows.

Warming Up

Warming up prepares your body for exercise in a number of ways. It does so by gradually increasing your heart rate, distributing blood to exercising muscles, warming the temperature of muscles, and improving circulation. Warming up decreases muscle soreness and decreases the risk of injury to muscles, tendons, ligaments and other connective tissues. Furthermore, warming up reduces muscles tightness and cramping.

To warmup for an aerobic activity, first walk around for a few minutes, and then perform slow stretches. Next, work at an intensity of *fairly light* on the RPE — Rating of Perceived Exertion Scale. Keep your target heart rate below your — THR — target heart rate range. Do this for at least five minutes. (RPE and THR range are discussed in later paragraphs.)

Cooling Down

Cooling down gradually decreases your heart rate, recirculates, and redistributes blood. It is very important that MVPers properly cool down after exercise.

When exercise is abruptly stopped without cooling down, blood tends to pool in muscles that were exercised. For example, if you were walking or biking, blood would pool in your legs. As blood pools, less blood recirculates throughout your body. MVPers tend to already have a lower blood volume, and therefore, less blood to circulate. Without proper cooling down, MVPers are more prone to lightheadedness, dizziness, and palpitations. Furthermore, cooling down decreases the risk of muscle soreness, injury, and fatigue. Therefore, cool down for a minimum of five to ten minutes. Perform your last exercise slowly. Do so at an RPE of *fairly light*. Example: If your last exercise is walking on a treadmill at 4.0 mph at a 5% grade, then walk at 0% and gradually decrease the speed. To finish, stretch the major muscle groups that you used.

Stretching

During your initial warmup and during the last part of your cool down, stretch all major muscles you either will use or did use in your workout activity. This must be done correctly.

To warm your muscles and maximize flexibility, walk for a few minutes prior to your warmup stretches. Hold each stretch for 10–20 seconds. Don't stretch beyond a feeling of a slight muscle pull. *Do not bounce.* Bouncing activates a muscular reflex — the stretch reflex. Instead of stretching, your muscles contract. Bouncing combined with contracting muscle can produce injury and soreness, and doesn't improve flexibility.

If you feel pain during the stretch, lessen the amount you are stretching. If pain persists, avoid that stretch. *Do not hold your breath* — breathe normally.

If your symptoms include lightheadedness or dizziness when standing up, avoid stretches that involve abrupt postural changes. These include: windmills and touching the floor from a standing position.

Examples of Warm Up and Cool Down Exercises

As you preform these stretches, hold the stretch to where you feel a slight pull in the muscle.

Do not bounce and do not hold your breath.

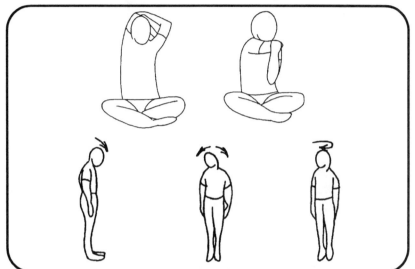

SHOULDER AND ARM STRETCHES

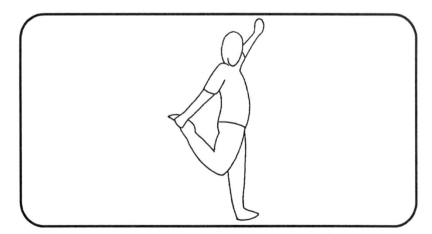

QUADRICEPS STRETCH: Pull your leg straight back until you feel a slight pull in your quadriceps — the muscles in front of your thigh. Variation: do the same by lying on your side.

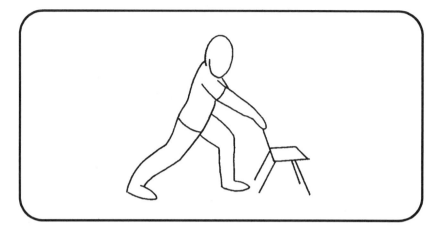

CALF STRETCH: Place one foot in front of the other. Point both feet straight forward, with your heels flat. Lunge forward with front leg bent and back leg straight.

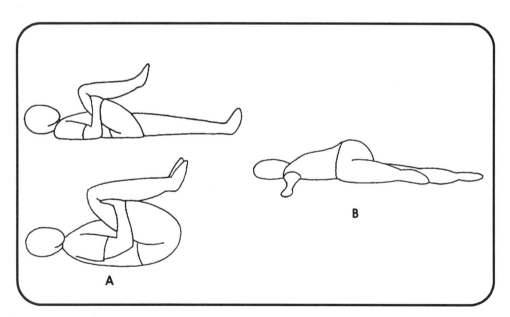

LOWER BACK STRETCHES: (A) Stretches lower back and gluteal — buttock — muscles.   (B) Stretches lower back and hip muscles.

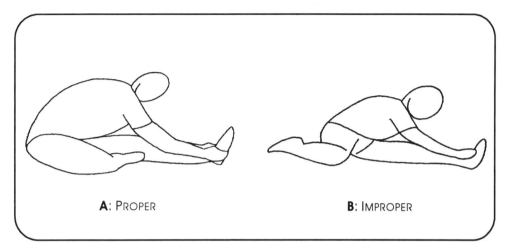

A: PROPER   B: IMPROPER

A. HAMSTRING STRETCH: Place one foot on the opposite knee. Keep your leg straight with foot pointed toward the ceiling. Bend forward from your waist till you feel a slight pull in your hamstrings — muscle on the back of your thigh.

B. IMPROPER HAMSTRING STRETCH: This can strain your knees.

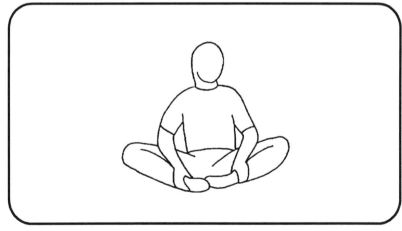

INNER LEG STRETCH

Exercises to Avoid with MVPS

Avoid exercises that involve abrupt postural changes such as the following.

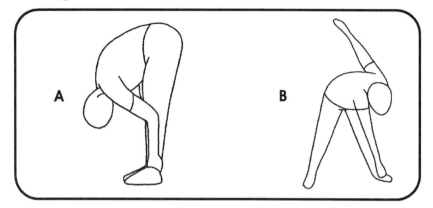

A. BENDING OVER TO TOUCH YOUR TOES.   B. WINDMILLS

Avoid activities requiring extreme exertion.

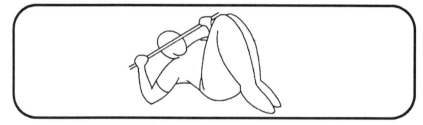

LIFTING HEAVY WEIGHTS.

Intensity

As one of the most important components of an exercise prescription — intensity means how *hard* you work. Age, fitness level and overall health status determine your level of intensity. To prescribe and monitor exercise intensity, various techniques are used. For example, two such methods are heart rate and rating of perceived exertion. These methods offer a guide for monitoring, and therefore controlling the intensity of exercise.

Optimal cardiovascular conditioning occurs when the intensity of exercise maintains a heart rate between 60% to 85% of a maximal heart rate — the target heart rate range. Cardiovascular improvements are *less* with exercise *below* a target rate. Exercising *above* a target range adds little or no improvement in the cardiovascular system, and places you at a greater risk of injury and MVPS symptoms.

Because MVPers often have inappropriate heart-rate responses to physical activity, a target heart-rate range may not be appropriate. To control exercise intensity, therefore, rely on a rating-of-perceived exertion — RPE Scale. The degree of overall effort exerted during exercise is rated on a scale of 1 to 10. A rating of 2 equates with exercise done easily and without strain. A rating of 10 means the exercise is so difficult you can't continue.

RATING OF PERCEIVED EXERTION SCALE	
1	Very, very easy
2	Very easy
3	Easy
4	
5	Somewhat hard
6	
7	Hard
8	Very hard
9	
10	Very, very hard

Some MVPers may wish to use a target heart rate — THR — range. Although a maximal graded exercise test gives a more accurate determination, there are other methods of calculating a THR range.

One method is to estimate your target heart rate range. First, subtract your age from 220 to determine your predicted *maximal* heart rate. For example, the age-predicted maximal heart rate for an MVPer of 30 years is 190 bpm — beats per minute. Next, determine your target heart rate *range*. Take 60 percent (.60) to 85 percent (.85) times your *maximal heart rate*. If you are 30, your target heart rate range is 114 to 162 beats per minute.

Another method, Karvonen's method, considers your RHR — resting heart rate — and is more accurate. To obtain RHR — your resting pulse rate — do so immediately before arising, when you are comfortable and rested. Then, enter your RHR into the following formula:

KARVONEN'S FORMULA

RHR = resting heart rate
MHR = maximum heart rate
(MHR – RHR) × .60 + RHR =
                    the lower end of your target heart rate range
(MHR – RHR) × .85 + RHR =
                    the upper end of your target heart rate range

For example, an MVPer of 30 years, with a resting heart rate of 70, age-predicted maximum heart rate — MHR — is 190 (220 – 30 = 190 bpm). Use these numbers with Karvonen's Formula to establish the target heart rate range at 142 to 172 bpm.

(MHR – RHR) × .60 + RHR
(190 – 70) × .60 + 70 = 142

(MHR – RHR) × .85 + RHR
(190 – 70) × .85 + 70 = 172

Therefore:

142 bpm (beats per minute) = lower end of target range
172 bpm (beats per minute) = upper end of target range

For exercise to be effective, the workout needs to be intense enough to maintain the heart rate within this range.

Obtaining Your Pulse Rate

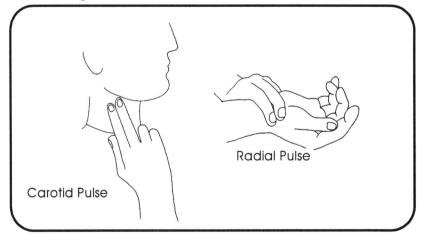

Radial Pulse

Carotid Pulse

(1) Carotid pulse: Place your index and middle finger lightly on your carotid artery. To find this artery locate your Adam's apple. Next, slide your fingers into the groove next to it. Press until you feel a steady pulse — be careful not to press hard.

OR

(2) Radial pulse: Place your index and middle fingers on the thumb side of the inside of your wrist to find your radial pulse.

Count your pulse for 10 seconds. Multiply this number by six. This gives your heart rate per minute.

When exercising, you should not feel dizzy, fatigued, breathless, or overexerted. Furthermore, you should not experience undue muscle pain or fatigue. One way to gauge your exercise intensity is your ability to converse with a friend. If you are huffing and puffing, barely able to speak, your exercise intensity is too hard. If, however, you can talk comfortably and the work feels somewhat challenging, you are working at the proper intensity. The proper intensity — working hard enough — equals a perceived exertion of *somewhat hard* on the RPE scale. If the exercise is too difficult, decrease your workload.

If the exercise is too easy, increase your workload. Remember: intense, unaccustomed activity often aggravates MVPS symptoms.

Type — Mode — of Exercise

Any activity that uses large muscle groups, is appropriate if it is rhythmic and aerobic, and is maintained at the proper intensity and duration. Exercise that meets these criteria include: walking, bicycling, rowing, jogging, cross-country skiing, aerobic dance, and swimming. *If you presently do not exercise on a regular basis, start with a low-intensity activity such as walking on a level surface.* As your fitness level improves, try other types of more intense activities such as aerobic dance, cross country skiing, or walking uphill.

Find an activity you enjoy. If you dislike biking, don't join a club with only bikes — you won't exercise. Combine types of activities. In addition to adding variety, you tone different muscle groups. Try different types of aerobic activity on different days. Do not assume, however, that because you are conditioned to one type of activity, you will be conditioned for others. Different exercises strengthen different muscles. This is known as training specificity. Unless you do a specific exercise regularly, your muscles may tire and become sore. If, therefore, you begin a new exercise, start slowly.

Types of Aerobic Exercise: Advantages, Disadvantages and Tips

Find one or more of the following that you enjoy, that fits your lifestyle, and that you tolerate. If you have trouble with your knees, ankles, hips, or back, stay with non-weightbearing activities — swimming or bicycling, or low-impact activities — walking, or low-impact aerobics.

Aerobic Dance

For people who like to exercise to music and like to exercise in groups, aerobic dance is perfect. Aerobic exercise combines calisthenics and dance steps with music. Compared with other forms of exercise, aerobic exercise is relatively inexpensive. You can take a class or rent a tape.

Two types of aerobic dance are: low-impact and high-impact aerobics. Low-impact requires one foot to always be on the ground. This reduces the stress on joints, and in turn, injury that sometimes occurs with traditional forms of aerobic dance. The intensity of low-impact aerobics varies from low to high, and depends upon the extent of exaggeration of the exercise movement. In other words, the more you move your arms and the higher you lift your legs, the greater the intensity of the workout.

High-impact aerobics involve running and jumping. This increases stress on joints, and the risk of injury. In fact, the forces incurred during high-impact aerobics can exceed three times your body weight. If you have back or joint problems, if you are overweight, or if high-impact aerobics causes pain, then low-impact aerobics are a better choice. If you tolerate and prefer high impact aerobics, limit this to every other day. This helps decrease the risk of injury.

If you don't exercise regularly, don't start with aerobics. Many MVPers experience undue fatigue when starting an aerobics class. Increase your fitness level first — start a walking program. When you can walk at a brisk pace for a minimum of 20 minutes, sign up for the class.

Before you enroll, make certain the instructor is qualified. Choose one who is certified by a reputable organization, one who is enthusiastic, and one who motivates you to regularly exercise.

Find a class that follows appropriate exercise guidelines including warming up and cooling down.

Work at you own pace — that's crucial. If the workout feels hard, do not exaggerate your movements — move your arms less, or not at all. Instead of running, march in place. Exercise to a perception of somewhat hard. Remember, avoid abrupt postural changes.

Be certain your body positions are correct. This avoids soreness and injury. Keep your feet and knees pointing in the same direction. When running in place or jumping, be sure to roll your feet from your heels to your toes. This helps prevent your calf muscles from getting sore, cramped, or injured. Most important, wear proper, well-fitting shoes. Avoid wearing running shoes. Because of the specificity of foot-impact mechanics, running shoes, along with most other athletic shoes, are not suitable for aerobic dance.

Aerobic Dance Shoes

Look for:

- Impact protection — especially midsole

- Good arch support

- A gradually sloping sole — not the steeper sloping sole found in running shoes

- Adequate toe and heel padding

- Breathable uppers

- Traction that prevents slipping, but doesn't grab the floor

- A sturdy saddle — sides of the shoe — that provides stability for side-to-side motions

- A heel counter — the cup at the back of the shoe that wraps around the heel of the shoe — for lateral stability to the heel area

- Flexibility

Air Bike

Not only does an air bike provide an excellent nonweight-bearing cardiovascular workout, it also tones your arm and leg muscles. Fan blades give the bike its air resistance. The faster you pedal, or the harder you pull, the greater the resistance. You can reach your target heart rate, or a perception of somewhat hard, easier with an air bike than with ordinary stationary bikes. Therefore, begin slowly.

Start by warming up at an intensity of *fairly light*, or at less than 1.0 Kilopond. Next, gradually increase the intensity. Alternate exercising your arms and legs. Rest your arms every other minute. This allows them to gradually adjust to the exercise. Continue to exercise to a perception of somewhat hard. If the exercise feels too intense, pedal slower. If the workload is too easy, pedal faster.

Avoid using *only* your arms, especially if you are deconditioned. Contracting muscles help pump the increased amount of blood needed during exercise. Arm exercise involves a smaller muscle mass than leg exercise. With arm exercise, less help is offered by the contracting muscle mass to pump blood throughout the body. To compensate, your heart rate increases. Therefore, exercise your arms and legs together — you're heart rate won't increase as rapidly. Remember, cool down the same way you warmed up.

In addition to upright bikes, air bikes are available in fully and semirecumbent positions. Recumbent bikes have a bucket seat, have pedals that are more in front — rather than directly underneath, and are more comfortable for those with low back pain.

Arm Ergometer

An arm ergometer is like a bike for your arms. While you are seated or standing, your arms spin a crank at varying speed and intensity. Arm ergometry is a good cardiovascular workout and it also tones your arms and shoulders. Most people, however, do not have the arm strength to maintain the intensity and duration required for an aerobic exercise session. Furthermore, arm work can cause an abrupt increase in heart rate.

Despite its difficulties, it is useful to add three to five minutes of arm ergometry to your workout. This helps strengthen your upper body and adds variety to your workout. For those who want to use only an arm ergometer, alternate rest periods with spinning the crank until you feel fatigued.

Although you can sit while cranking the arm ergometer, it is best to stand and move your legs. Standing and moving counters gravitational forces, avoids blood pooling in your legs, and promotes recirculation of blood. This is particularly important for MVPers with symptoms of dizziness or lightheadedness.

To exercise, begin by turning the intensity knob to zero resistance. Set the timer for two or three minutes. Position yourself at a comfortable proximity to the arm crank. Begin turning it at a speed of 50 revolutions per minute. Gradually increase the speed. If you feel any discomfort, slow down the cranking speed.

Bicycle Ergometer

Bicycle ergometers — stationary bicycles — are nonweight-bearing, tone leg and buttock muscles and give you a cardiovascular workout. If you are deconditioned, a stationary bike is a good first choice. You can exercise at low-to-moderate intensities. A disadvantage, however, is that your legs will fatigue before you achieve your target heart rate. To reduce leg fatigue, decrease the resistance and increase pedal speed. As your cardiovascular fitness improves, move to a higher-intensity exercise that you can perform without being limited by leg fatigue. If you have access to both a standard stationary bicycle and an air bike, progress to an air bike after a few weeks of using the stationary bicycle. For further comfort and lower back support, use a recumbent bike.

To help pass the time while riding a stationary bike, work out with a friend, exercise to music, or exercise watching television. You might want to buy an inexpensive magazine stand, attach it to your bicycle, and read while you ride.

The stationary bike seat must be properly adjusted. To do this, stand next to the bike and adjust the seat so it's approximately at hip level. Next, climb on the bicycle and put the balls of your feet on the pedals. When each pedal reaches its lowest point in the cycle, your leg should be slightly bent — almost straight — you should not strain to reach the pedal.

To adjust the tension, first remove all tension from the bicycle wheel by adjusting the appropriate knob. Next, begin pedaling. You can't accurately adjust the tension till you pedal at your workout speed. Pedal at 50–60 revolutions per minute. Follow the guidelines in this chapter for details about duration, intensity, frequency, progression, and proper warmup and cool down.

Warm up with little to no intensity — about 0 to 20 watts per 50–60 rpm — revolutions per minute. Next, continue to pedal at 50 to 60 rpm. Gradually increase the tension till the work feels "Somewhat Hard." After your workout, decrease the tension and cool down.

Bicycling Outside

Outdoor bicycling is easy to learn and gives you the opportunity to sightsee. It is nonweight-bearing, can be performed at a low-to-high intensity, and requires only a sturdy bicycle and comfortable clothing. To be safe, especially if riding near automobile traffic, invest in a bicycle helmet. Prices for bicycles vary from a standard, inexpensive bike to an expensive, deluxe racer. Before you buy, compare prices. Check cyclists' magazines or *Consumer Reports*. Ask a reputable bicycle dealer or experienced cyclists for advice.

Dress for comfort and protection from the weather. Wear shoes with heavy soles, and wool or cotton socks. Tuck shoe laces in, and secure pants cuffs so they don't get caught in the chain. If you plan on biking regularly, invest in a pair of shoes made specifically for biking.

Although rain or snow may prevent you from cycling outside, you can buy rollers or indoor trainers for indoor riding. Cycling on rollers or indoor trainers mimics your outdoor bicycle workout better than riding a stationary bike.

Proper frame size and bicycle seat, as well as proper handlebar adjustment are important for comfort and safety. As you stand in bare feet, the bicycle frame size should be nine to ten inches less than your inseam measurement. The inseam measurement is the distance between your crotch and the floor. Because of variations such as tire size, this formula doesn't always hold true. Therefore, always straddle the bike you intend to buy. Then — barefoot, with both feet flat on the floor, be certain the top tube of the frame is 3/4" to 1" below your crotch.

Sit on the bike. Then, adjust the seat's height.

Next, center your heel on a pedal at its lowest point in the cycle.

With your pelvis level on the seat, fully extend your legs.

To ride, pedal on your toes and slightly bend your knees. Your leg should be fully extended while your pelvis is level on the seat. For information about any other adjustments, ask a salesperson, or refer to the handbook.

To begin your workout, ride on a flat surface and use low gear. Keep the intensity *fairly light* for five to ten minutes. Pedal continuously at a comfortable pace. Usually, the pedal speed is faster than a stationary bike — about 70–90 rpm on an outdoor bicycle versus 50–60 rpm on a bicycle ergometer. Increase the intensity to *somewhat hard*. To do this, increase the gear, pedal faster, or ride up a hill. Remember, you want to ride continuously for 30 to 40 minutes. Coasting does not count. Cool down the same way you warmed up.

Cross-country Skiing

Cross-country skiing is an all-around exercise — it combines hiking and skiing. It is low impact and uses both arms and legs rhythmically and continuously making it an excellent source of cardiovascular conditioning. Cross-country skiing also tones all of the major muscles and muscle groups.

While good weather conditions are needed to ski outside, there are cross-country-ski simulators for indoor use. If you buy one, make certain the skis glide smoothly, and there is an intensity adjustment for both arms and the legs.

Cross-country skiing requires a lot of cardiovascular endurance, muscular strength, and coordination — *it is not for people starting to get into shape.* The intensity of cross-country skiing is such that it is difficult for most people to endure for a complete exercise session. Therefore, if you are beginning an exercise program, first get into shape. Start with lower-intensity activities such as walking or biking. Then, gradually add a few minutes of cross-country-ski simulator activity to your workout. Alternate intervals of three-to-five minute rest periods as you exercise on the ski simulator. Gradually increase your workout time. Use the cross-country-ski simulator for the entire workout, or alternate the ski simulator with periods of a lower-intensity exercise.

If the ski simulator has a support pad, adjust it to hip level. Press lightly against the pad when cross-country skiing, but keep your weight on your feet — not on the pad. Move your legs back and forth until you get your balance. Keep your knees slightly bent and use a comfortable stride. With the toes of one foot, push one ski back, and keep your other foot flat as it glides forward. Once you feel comfortable using only your legs, add your arms. Alternate each arm forward with the opposite leg. If your right arm is forward, then your left leg is forward. Swing your arms like pendulums — extend your arm until your elbow is straight. Cross-country skiing takes coordination and lots of patience to master.

Jogging

Jogging is inexpensive, lets you enjoy the outdoors, and offers excellent cardiovascular conditioning. Jogging, however, is associated with a higher risk of injury than other nonweight-bearing or low-impact activities. It places the stress of three times your body weight on your joints, your back, and rest of your body. If you are overweight or have trouble with your knees, ankles, hips or back, don't jog. Swimming — a nonweight-bearing activity, or walking — a low-impact exercise — is preferable.

If you prefer to jog and are able, do so *no more* than *every other day*. This reduces your risk of injury. If you want to exercise daily, perform a nonweight-bearing or low-impact activity on alternate days. Before you start, choose a good running shoe. Make sure there is at least 1/2 to 3/4 of an inch between your toes and the front of the shoe. Choose one with sturdy arch support and a durable sole. Be certain the sole is a good shock absorber. To minimize up-and-down, or side-to-side heel movement, select a shoe with a firm, well-fitting heel counter — a cup at the back of the shoe that wraps around the heel for reinforcement.

For those beginning to exercise, start with a walking program. When you can walk briskly for a half hour, try a combination of walking and jogging. Do this for about twenty minutes. For example, start with repeated intervals of walking two minutes, then walking and jogging thirty seconds. Gradually *increase* the length of the jogging intervals, and *decrease* the length of the walking intervals. Do this till you can continuously jog for 20–30 minutes. Remember to warm up before, and to cool down after. For example, walk or slowly jog for five to ten minutes both before and after your jog.

Develop an appropriate running style to maximize jogging efficiency and comfort, as well as to prevent injuries and soreness. Make certain you land on your heel, and roll off of the ball of your foot. Breathe normally through your mouth and nose; relax your arms and shoulders. Ask an experienced runner, athletic trainer, or other sports-medicine professional to check your running style and correct serious errors.

Rowing

Rowing, an excellent source of cardiovascular exercise, tones most of the major muscle groups with little stress on your joints. Rowing, however is not a good choice if you have back or knee problems. Because rowing is a more intense exercise and difficult to perform for an entire workout, use the rower for only a few minutes as part of your workout.

If you are beginning an exercise program, do not start with rowing. First, perform less intense cardiovascular activities to develop cardiovascular fitness.

Properly use the rowing machine to maximize cardiovascular conditioning and to decrease your risk of injury and back strain.

As you pull back with your arms, push back with your legs. Initially, keep your hands facing downward — overhanded. At times, row underhanded — hands facing upward — to strengthen your biceps. Do not extend your legs to the point that your knees lock.

Next, slide forward. Repeat this cycle rhythmically. Keep your back straight and perpendicular to the floor throughout the rowing cycle. If you feel any discomfort in your back, or other part of your body, make sure that your rowing technique is correct. If you still experience discomfort, then discontinue rowing as a component of your fitness program.

To begin, warm up for three to five minutes; adjust the resistance to the lowest level; and row at a speed that feels *fairly light*. For your first few sessions, the warm-up period adequately accustoms your body to this piece of equipment. Later on, increase the intensity of your workout until it feels *somewhat hard*. To do this, increase the resistance, or increase the speed. In general, a good pace is 20 to 25 strokes per minute. When you finish, cool down for five minutes at the same intensity you warmed up.

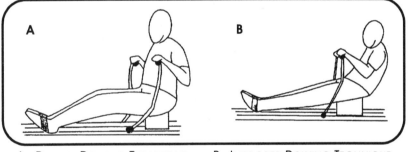

A. PROPER ROWING TECHNIQUE   B. IMPROPER ROWING TECHNIQUE

Stair Machine

A stair machine provides a very good low-impact, cardiovascular workout. It works all of the major muscles in the lower part of your body: muscles in your legs, hips, and buttocks. If, however, you have weak ankles, knees, or quadriceps, a stair machine may not be your best choice.

It is best to first strengthen weakened ankles, knees, or quads with other lower-intensity aerobic activity.

Intensity on a stair machine is a function of step height, stepping speed, and the resistance you work against. To start, first adjust the resistance to a low level. Next, adjust the step height to 6 or 8 inches. Increase and decrease the intensity of your workout by the stepping speed. Follow the previously described guidelines for warming up, working out, and cooling down.

If you experience discomfort in your knees, ankles, or elsewhere while using a stair machine, make sure the step height is not adjusted too high. If this does not correct the problem, then stop using stair machines.

Swimming

Swimming, an excellent source of cardiovascular conditioning, is nonweight-bearing, and can tone all of the major muscle groups in your body. Because your body weight is supported by water, swimming is less stressful on your joints than most activities. Therefore, the risk of injuries in swimming versus high-impact activities is much lower.

The energy cost of swimming is about four times that of running an equal distance. While energy is needed for your arms and legs to propel you through the water, energy must also be expended to keep you afloat. The drag of the water also provides excellent resistance that improves muscular strength and endurance.

As compared with someone who does the same amount of work and achieves the same cardiovascular benefits with land sports, the swimmer's heart rate will be lower. In fact, studies show that when someone swims, his maximum heart rate averages 13 beats per minute less than it would on land. Therefore, if you use a target heart rate to monitor the intensity of exercise, subtract 13 from your actual, or your age-predicted maximum heart rate before using it in Karvonen's Equation.

To warm up, swim slowly for 5 to 10 minutes at an intensity that feels *fairly light*. Then, swim more briskly for 20 to 30 minutes at an intensity that feels *somewhat hard*. To finish, swim slowly for 5 to 10 minutes to cool down. As part of your warmup or cool down, you may hold on to the edge of the pool and gently kick your legs.

Walking

Walking requires no special skill and, except for a good pair of walking shoes, no special equipment. It is an excellent activity for people starting to get into shape, as well as for experienced athletes. Furthermore, while walking puts the stress of *one and one-quarter times* your weight on your joints and back, jogging puts approximately *three times* your weight on your body.

A good pair of walking shoes maximizes safety, comfort, and enjoyment. Look for shoes with more flexibility than a running shoe — ones that have extra shock protection at the heel — the focus of impact. Choose ones that have good arch support to absorb shock that would otherwise be transmitted to you body. Be sure the shoe is durable, with a stiff toe box, a breathable upper (top of the shoe), and with plenty of space between your toes and the front of the shoe.

As you get into shape, increase the intensity of your workout. Increase your walking pace; swing your arms more; walk uphill; or add light wrist weights — two pounds or less per arm.

Walking Outside

Walking outside is enjoyable and beneficial. It allows you to explore the outdoors while you become physically fit. Too, you may socialize and make new friends through noncompetitive walking clubs — such as Volksmarching Clubs — and organizational-sponsored walks for charity. To walk with a friend or with a group also motivates you to continue your fitness program.

If the weather is bad, continue to walk at a mall or at a fitness center[1] for a good reason. Suppose you are now in shape physically from first walking on a flat surface. It's time to increase the *intensity* of your exercise program. Why? After a few weeks of conditioning, your cardiovascular system gets stronger. Now, it takes a higher degree of intensity to both increase your heart rate and to feel that the exercise is *somewhat hard*.

How can you do this? Increase your walking pace to a fast, comfortable pace. If the exercise still doesn't feel *somewhat hard*, wear one- or two-pound wrist weights and swing your arms more. Should this strain your shoulders, don't use the weights. Furthermore, don't add ankle weights. They place added stress on your joints and back. Rather, to increase intensity, walk up some hills.

Walking in the Mall

Walking in a local shopping mall offers a free, often convenient alternative to walking outside. It has the advantage of offering shelter from rain, snow, and extremes of temperature. Many shopping malls keep hallways open both before the shops open,

---

[1]Some fitness centers let you pay on a single-session basis.

and after they close. Mall-walkers' clubs offer group support, camaraderie, and instruction. Contact you local chapter of the American Heart Association for helpful information. Determine which local malls welcome walkers; what is the mileage of the various local malls; and which local malls support walking organizations.

Again, remember to increase the *intensity* of your walk. Increase your walking speed. If necessary, wear one-to-two pound wrist weights. Then, vigorously swing your arms.

Walking on a Treadmill

Walking on a treadmill offers a more controlled workout intensity. By increasing its grade or slant, you achieve the same intensity as a jog. But, unlike a jog, you add no stress to your joints. Walking on a treadmill, does not tone any muscles in your arms. To get a complete workout, add arm work such as using light, free weights or using an air bike.

Proper use of a treadmill is necessary for maximum safety and to achieve cardiovascular benefits. First, before you turn on the treadmill put *one foot on either side of the conveyer belt*. Turn on the power and the conveyor belt. Then, adjust the speed. If you are out of shape and don't know what speed to start with, begin at 1.5 mph. Tap one foot on the belt to get a feel for the speed of the treadmill. Begin to walk on the treadmill. Take comfortable strides. Keep your hips under your shoulders; keep your arms and shoulders relaxed; and keep your body near the front of the treadmill. Walk heel to toe. Experiment till you find a speed that feels *fairly light* and warm up for five minutes. Gradually work up to an intensity that feels *somewhat hard*.

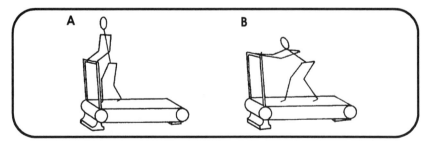

A. CORRECT POSITION. Walk erectly near front of belt, hand(s) resting on handrail or at your side.

B. INCORRECT POSITION. Walking bent over hanging onto handrail for support.

Gradually work up to your fastest speed with which you're comfortable. Once this no longer feels *somewhat hard*, gradually increase the grade or slant of the treadmill by 2% to 3%. Walk for at least two minutes at each increase in the grade. During your last 5–10 minutes, gradually decrease both the grade and speed of the treadmill. Don't get off till the treadmill is flat and the belt hardly moves.

Finally, turn off the treadmill; step off, but keep moving. Continue your cool down. Walk slowly for a few minutes. You may feel slightly dizzy when you step off a treadmill because your body develops a forward momentum without actually moving forward. When you stop, your body retains some of this momentum. Some MVPers experience more dizziness. If you stop to catch your balance, the problem worsens. Blood has already pooled in the legs. By standing still, gravitational forces further cause blood to pool in the legs. This lowers blood pressure in the upper body and causes more dizziness. Dizziness decreases once you cool down and walk around for a few minutes.

Frequency of Exercise

Regular exercise is an important component of a fitness program. For MVPS symptom control, schedule exercise at least three times a week on alternate days. Although daily exercise doesn't harm the cardiovascular system, it can put excess stress on your joints. Therefore, limit high-impact activities — jogging or jumping — to alternate days.

Duration and Progression of Training

Your present level of fitness determines the initial duration of your exercise session. While some MVPers start with 30 minutes of exercise, others barely make ten. Either way, ten minutes of exercise is better than zero minutes of exercise.

If you begin an aerobic exercise program, start with 10 to 20 minutes of exercise. Add two to five minutes each session until you reach 30 to 45 minutes. This time *does not* include warmup and cool down.

Overall improvement depends upon your initial level of fitness — the lower your fitness, the greater the improvement. Adjust your exercise prescription as improvements in fitness and conditioning occur. Once you achieve cardiovascular conditioning — maintain it.

SIGNS OF IMPROVEMENT

Signs that regular aerobic exercise is increasing the efficiency of your cardiorespiratory system include:

- A lower resting heart rate

- A lower heart rate while doing the same amount of work

- A post-exercise heart rate that more quickly than before approaches your normal daily activities

- An increase in your endurance during exercise and normal daily activities

- A decrease in the intensity and frequency of MVPS

Exercise Prescription: Muscular Fitness

Aerobic exercise is the most important type of exercise for someone with MVPS. But, do *add* exercises that develop muscular tone, strength, and endurance. Take special care to properly perform these exercises, and thereby avoid aggravating MVPS symptoms.

Many women worry that lifting weights develops large, bulging muscles. In fact, women get much less hypertrophy — increase in muscle size — than men do. Change in muscle size is mediated by the hormone testosterone — present in much lower levels in women.

PRINCIPLES TO CONSIDER WHEN DEVELOPING A WEIGHT TRAINING PROGRAM

- Overload
- Progressive resistance
- Specificity
- Arrangement of exercises
- Frequency
- Duration
- Safety

Principles of Strength Training

Consider the following principles as you develop a strength training program.

(1) *Overload Principle*: To strengthen a muscle, it needs to work against more resistance, or lift more weight than usual.

(2) *Progressive Resistance Principle*: To reach your desired level of strength and endurance, gradually increase the amount of resistance applied. To maintain this level of muscular strength and endurance, continue to lift the same amount of weight.

(3) *Specificity Principle:* The development of muscular fitness is specific to the muscle group exercised, the type of contraction, and the intensity of exercise. In other words, weight-training programs should exercise muscles you actually use in sports or in everyday activities. They should also mimic both the movement patterns and intensities involved.

(4) *Principle of Arrangement of Exercises:* To achieve maximum benefit from a training session, exercise your larger muscles before your smaller ones. Smaller muscles aid larger muscles. If you first exercise the smaller muscles, they will fatigue. Consequently, this limits the amount of weight the larger muscles and muscle groups can lift. Similarly, arrange training programs so no two successive exercises involve the same muscle or muscle group.

EXERCISE MUSCLE GROUPS IN THE FOLLOWING ORDER	
First	Upper legs and hips
Second	Chest and upper arms
Third	Back and posterior legs
Fourth	Lower legs and ankles
Fifth	Shoulders and posterior upper arms
Sixth	Abdomen
Seventh	Anterior upper arms

Type of Strength Training Exercise

Strength training exercises include: isometric, isotonic, and isokinetic. For MVPers, the most appropriate is *isotonic* exercise. Isotonic exercises include sit ups, crunches, using a weight station, and lifting free weights — hand weights or barbells.

Intensity

(**Caution:** If you note an increase in MVPS symptoms, try lighter weights. Then, if you still can't tolerate weight lifting, stop. Do other types of exercise.)

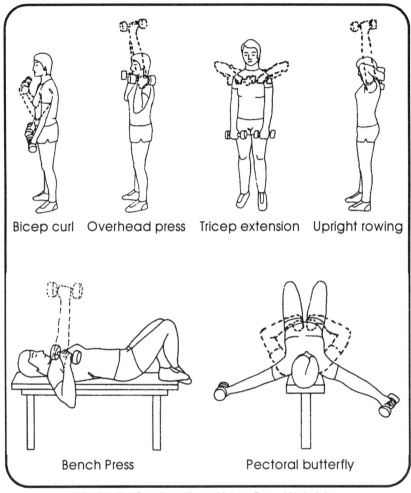

Bicep curl Overhead press Tricep extension Upright rowing

Bench Press Pectoral butterfly

Isotonic Contractions Using Free Weights

To lift weights, start with ones that are easy to lift, and ones you can comfortably lift at least eight times. Women: try two to five pounds. Men: try five to ten pounds. To increase muscular endurance, gradually increase the repetitions — the number of times a weight is lifted without a rest. Add one or two repetitions per exercise session till you lift the weight 15 times. Then, you can increase the weight.

How much weight you lift depends on your tolerance of the weight, your fitness level, and the types of your daily activities. An exercise physiologist, sports medicine physician, or physical therapist can help determine your weight limit. In general, female MVPers can gradually work up to 20 to 30 pounds without an increase in symptoms. Many male MVPers tolerate even higher weights. Remember, start out with light weights, and increase weights *gradually*. Decrease the weight if you note an increase in symptoms.

Frequency

Studies show that muscles respond best after a day of rest. Why? Part of the muscle strengthening process involves partially tearing down muscle tissue and rebuilding stronger tissue. Therefore, perform muscular resistance exercises only two to three, nonconsecutive days per week.

Duration

The duration equals the amount of time it takes to perform the prescribed number of repetitions and sets — groups of repetitions that alternate with rest periods. Duration is more important with cardiovascular exercise than with weight-resistance exercise.

Additional How To's

Always consult your physician before starting a weight training program.

Warmup before you lift weights. First, stretch the muscles that you will use. Next, perform the same movements that you will do while lifting weights. Do this with either a light weight or no weight for a few repetitions.

Never hold your breath when exercising. As you lift a weight, *slowly exhale* to prevent a spike in blood pressure. Slowly perform this initial movement to the count of two. Let the weight down slowly to the count of four. The movement of letting the weight down produces most of the strength-building benefits. Therefore, do this slowly.

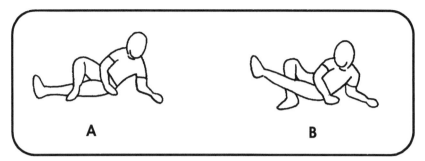

A. Proper Adductor Lift (Inner Thigh Lift)
B. Improper Adductor Lift (Inner Thigh Lift)

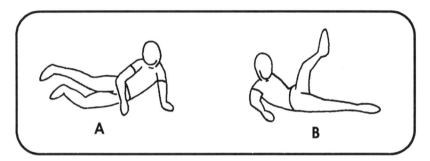

A. Proper Abductor Lift (Outer Thigh Lift)
B. Improper Abductor Lift (Outer Thigh Lift)

Crunches Versus Sit Ups

During the first few degrees of a sit up you use your abdominal muscles. Then, you use the muscles in your back which may lead to back strain. A better way to strengthen your abdominal muscles, is with a *crunch* — a modified sit up.

To do a crunch:

5. Lie on the floor with knees bent, feet flat, and arms crossed over your chest.

6. As you lift your upper body by contracting your abdominal muscles, leave your lower back flat on the floor. Exhale as you lift up.

7. Lift no more than a 30- to 45-degree angle.

8. To a *slow* count of four, inhale as you lower your upper body to the floor.

To prevent neck strain, lift only with your abdominal muscles. Let your head come up with the rest of your body. To help prevent lower back strain, always keep your legs bent. Do not hook your feet under a bar or piece of furniture — otherwise, your hips and legs do most of the work. To work the sides of the abdominal area more effectively, add a slight twist to some of your crunches. Move each shoulder towards an opposite leg.

Start with five to ten crunches. Add one or two crunches per session till you work up to 20 to 30. If you tolerate them, you can perform up to 45 crunches. Divide these into three sets of 15 repetitions with brief periods of rest in between. Doing more will not be helpful. To make them more of a challenge, perform the crunches more slowly.

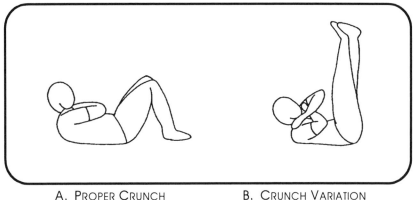

A. PROPER CRUNCH   B. CRUNCH VARIATION

Weight Station

A weight station is a piece of equipment with which you can work all of the major muscles and muscle groups in your body. Consult a sports-medicine professional for guidelines on the proper use of this equipment.

General Exercise Tips

When Should You Eat and Drink Relative to Exercise?

Never exercise immediately after you have eaten. Allow at least one hour after a light snack and two hours after a regular meal.

Be sure to replace the extra fluids lost during exercise. Drink plenty of water before, during, and after exercise. During heavy exercise, replace fluids with six to eight ounces of water every 15 minutes.

Unless you have high blood pressure, or your physician recommends that you reduce your sodium intake, use salt freely. The electrolytes in your food generally replace those lost during exercise except during prolonged, intense events such as marathons. Unless the event is over 90 minutes long, only water needs to be consumed during exercise.

What Should You Wear?

Wear proper athletic shoes along with breathable, cotton socks to both reduce the risk of blisters, and to absorb moisture. Wear loose-fitting, comfortable clothing. Choose cotton or wool fabrics because they allow skin to breathe. There are also several breathable, man-made fabrics such as lycra, Gore-Tex — waterproof, polypropylene, and coolmax. Wear layers to avoid the effects of wind and cold. Consult with sales representatives at reputable sporting-goods stores, or sports-medicine professionals, or refer to related literature for further information.

When Should You either Avoid or Lessen the Intensity of Exercise?

Avoid exercise if you don't feel well. Cold, fever, infection, diarrhea, or vomiting increase the metabolic demands of your body and increase your heart rate. Similarly, if you are tired, hot, have a slight cold or allergies, decrease the intensity and duration of your workout.

Avoid exercising in extremely warm — above 90 degrees and 80% humidity, or cold — below 32-degree weather. Decrease the intensity if you exercise in temperatures between 80 and 89 degrees. If you stay within the guidelines for RPE — Rating of Perceived Exertion scale, you automatically adhere to these temperature-and-illness guidelines.

What if You Experience Symptoms during Exercise?

If you experience symptoms, such as: palpitations, excessive fatigue, chest pain, or discomfort, excessive shortness of breath, or any unusual symptom, decrease your level of intensity. If the symptoms persist, cool down and stop exercising.

What if You Want to Buy Some Exercise Equipment?

Before you buy any exercise equipment, be sure you'll use it. Often times it soon becomes a dust collector. Many people become motivated by taking a fitness class, by joining a fitness club, or by exercising with a friend. Before you invest, experiment. Either use a friend's equipment or find a fitness facility that will let you try out different pieces of equipment. See what your body tolerates, and what you enjoy.

Once you decide upon a piece of equipment, try to get one that is used or in good repair. But, before you buy, try it out to make sure the equipment is sturdy, in good repair, and easy to operate.

For tips about advantages and disadvantages of specific types of exercise, exercise equipment, and how to use it, refer to "Types of Exercise."

What about Performing Activities in High Altitude?

Physical performance is reduced at high altitudes and may be particularly bothersome for MVPers who enjoy hiking, or skiing in the mountains. Subjective feelings of fatigue may be more pronounced than at sea level. Also, the heart may beat faster and feel more forceful.

To avoid this uncomfortable sensation, maintain a slower tempo. Perform the activity at a reduced intensity for less time. Don't push beyond a perception of *somewhat hard*. It takes longer at higher altitudes than at sea level to recover from intense activity. Remember to drink plenty of fluids prior to, during, and after your trip.

What about Participating in Athletic Sports Activities?

Sports activities include everything from auto racing to water polo, and individual clinical situations vary. *Participating in athletic sports, therefore, should be discussed with your physician* In general, your physician considers the degree of mitral regurgitation — back flow of blood flow into the left atrium, presence and type of arrhythmias, size of the heart chambers, your clinical history, your symptoms, and type of sports activity.

Myths about Exercise

No pain, no gain: Pain is a warning sign that you need to back off. You risk injury or an increase in symptoms if you continue. Warm up; cool down properly; don't intensely work out, and follow the guidelines discussed. You shouldn't have pain.

I can spot reduce fat from certain areas of my body: You can't spot reduce fat. You lose fat by burning more calories than you consume. Where you lose fat depends on your sex and your heredity. While exercises like sit ups or crunches strengthen and tone muscles, they don't spot reduce fat.

Exercise turns fat into muscle: Although aerobic exercise burns fat, and both weight-resistance and aerobic exercise improve muscle tone, they don't turn fat to muscle. For example, consider the big, muscular football player who becomes fat. He's accustomed to consuming enough calories to support an active, young body. As he gets older, he no longer remains physically active. His muscles atrophy — weaken and shrink in size — from lack of exercise. To top this off, he still eats as usual. Because he consumes more calories than he burns, he gets fat.

I am too old to start exercising: You are never too old to start exercising. Thousands of people in their 60's, 70's, and 80's begin exercise programs. It's inspiring to consider the tremendous gains in fitness they achieve.

I don't have enough energy to exercise: This is all the more reason to exercise. Within a few weeks exercise increases energy levels. Start slowly; be patient; and enjoy the results.

I don't have enough time to exercise: Make time. You'll find that regular cardiovascular exercise increases alertness, promotes self confidence, and increases energy levels. You may find, therefore, you become more efficient and accomplish more tasks with less fatigue. Ask yourself, "Am I worth giving up only three hours a week to better condition myself?"

Housework, golf, bowling, and chasing after small children is enough exercise: These activities can be tiring. They can improve flexibility. They can improve muscular strength. But, they don't meet the criteria for aerobic exercise. They don't provide benefits that cardiovascular exercises do.

Exercise will always increase your appetite: If you are normal weight and begin an exercise program, your appetite may increase slightly to compensate for the extra calories that you burn. If you are overweight and begin an exercise program, the exercise may actually help your body regulate your appetite.

Walking a mile quickly will burn more calories than walking a mile slowly: Regardless of how quickly or how slowly you walk a mile, you burn about the same number of calories. Of course, if you walk a mile quickly, you burn the calories faster — you burn more calories per hour — not per mile.

Passive exercise helps burn calories and helps you get stronger without the work: Passive exercise, such as riding on an electrically operated bicycle, may improve flexibility. It doesn't give you aerobic or muscle-toning exercise. To strengthen muscles, you have to work against a resistance. Remember, whichever one does the work — the machine or you — gets the benefits.

References

American College of Sports Medicine. 1991. *Guidelines for Exercise Testing and Prescription.* 4th edit. Lea & Febiger. Philadelphia.

American College of Sports Medicine. 1988. *Resource Manual for Guidelines for Exercise Testing and Prescription.* Lea & Febiger. Philadelphia.

Astrand, Per Olof & Rodahl, K. 1986. *Textbook of Work Physiology.* McGraw-Hill Book Co. New York.

Baumgartner, R., Chumlea, C, & Roche A. 1990. "Bioelectric impedance for body composition." In: *Exercise and Sport Sciences Reviews* (K. Pandolf & J. Holloszy, Eds.). Williams & Wilkins. Baltimore. 193–224.

Boudoulas, H., & Wooley, C. 1988. "Mitral valve prolapse: Childhood, pregnancy, athletics, and aviation." In: *Mitral Valve Prolapse and the Mitral Valve Prolapse Syndrome* (H. Boudoudas & C. Wooley, Eds.). Futura Publishers, Inc. Mount Kisco, New York. 609–631.

Borg, G. 1970. "Perceived exertion as an indicator of somatic stress." *Scandinavian Journal of Rehabilitative Medicine.* 2–3, 92–98.

Fletcher, C. 1984. *The Complete Walker.* Alfred A. Knopf, Inc. New York.

Fox, E. L., Kirby, T. E., & Fox, A. R. 1987. *Bases of Fitness.* Macmillan Publ. Co. New York.

Francis, L. L., Francis, P. R., & Welshons-Smith, K. 1985. "Aerobic dance injuries: a survey of instructors." *The Physician and Sportsmedicine.* **13:** (2).

Froelicher, V. 1987. *Exercise and the Heart: Clinical Concepts.*

2nd edit. Year Book Publishers, Inc. Chicago

Fontana, M., Wooley, C., Leighton, R., & Lewis, R. 1975. "Postural changes in left ventricular and mitral valvular dynamics in the systolic click-late systolic murmur syndrome." *Circulation.* **51**: 165–173.

Graves, J., Pollock, M., Montain, S., Jackson, A., & O'Keefe, J. 1987. "The effect of hand-held weights on the physiological responses to walking exercise." *Medicine and Science in Sports and Exercise.* **19:** (3) 260–265.

Graves, J. Martin, A., Miltenberger, L., & Pollock, M. 1988. "Physiological responses to walking with hand weights, wrist weights, and ankle weights." *Medicine and Science in Sports and Exercise.* **20:** (3), 265–271.

Guyton, A. C. 1996. *Textbook of Medical Physiology.* 7th edit. W. B. Saunders Co. Philadelphia.

Health Letter Associates. 1988, December. "The best all-around exercise." *University of California, Berkeley Wellness Letter.* **5:** (3) 6.

Health Letter Associates. 1987, March. "Swimming to a different beat." *University of California, Berkeley Wellness Letter.* **3:** (6) 7.

Health Letter Associates. 1990, May. "What if you did 5,000 sit-ups a month?" *University of California, Berkeley Wellness Letter.* **6**(8) 6.

Holland, H. J., Hoffmann, J. J., Vincent, W., Mayers, M., & Caston, A. 1990. "Treadmill vs steptreadmill ergometry." *The Physician and Sportsmedicine.* **18:** (1) 79–85.

Iskandrian, A. S. 1988. "Exercise left ventricular performance in patients with mitral valve prolapse." Urban & Vogel, **13:** (4) 243–248. Herz, Philadelphia.

Jackson, A. S., & Pollock, M. L. 1978. "Generalized equations for predicting body density of men." *British Journal of Nutrition.* **40**: 497–507.

Jackson, A. S., Pollock, M. L., & Ward, A. 1980. "Generalized equations for predicting body density of women." *Medicine in science, sports, & exercise.* **12**: 175–182.

Koszuta, L. E. 1987. "Can fitness be found at the top of the stairs?" *The Physician and Sportsmedicine.* **15:** (2) 165–169.

Lamb, D. 1984. *Physiology of Exercise: Responses and Adaptations.* Macmillan Publishing Co. New York.

Loften, M., Boileau, R., Massey, B., & Lohman, T. 1988. "Effect of arm training on central and peripheral circulatory function." *Medicine and Science in Sports and Exercise.* **20:** (2) 136–141.

Maresh, C. & Noble, B. 1984. "Utilization of perceived exertion ratings during exercise testing and training." In: *Cardiac Rehabilitation: Exercise Testing and Prescription* (L.K. Hall, Ed.). Spectrum Publications, Inc. 155–173.

Marino, J., May, L., & Bennett, H. 1981. *John Marino's Bicycling Book.* J. P. Tarcher, Inc. Los Angeles.

Maron, B. & Mitchell, J. 1994. "26th Bethesda Conference: Recommendations for determining eligibility for competition in athletes with cardiovascular abnormalities." *Journal of the American College of Cardiology.* **24**: 845–899.

Monahan, T. 1988. "Perceived exertion: an old exercise tool finds new applications." *The Physician and Sportsmedicine.* **16**: 174–179.

Nieman, D. 1986. *The Sports Medicine Fitness Course.* Bull Publishing Co. Palo Alto, California.

Pollock, M., & Mason, D. 1986. *Heart Disease and Rehabilitation.* 2nd edit. John Wiley & Sons. New York.

President's Council on Physical Fitness and Sports. 1971. Physical Fitness Research Digest. Series 1, No. 1. Washington, DC.

Rosiello, R., Mahler, D., & Ward, J. 1987. "Cardiovascular responses to rowing." *Medicine and Science in Sports and Exercise.* **19:** (3) 239–245.

Scordo, K. 1991. "Effects of aerobic exercise in symptomatic women with mitral valve prolapse." *American Journal of Cardiology.* **67**: 863–868.

Skinner, J., Hutsler, R., Bergsteinova, V., & Buskirk, E. 1973. "The validity and reliability of a rating scale of perceived exertion." *Medicine and Science in Sports.* **5:** (2) 94–96.

Wilmoth, S. 1986. *Leading Aerobic-Dance Exercise.* Human Kinetics Publishers, Inc. Champaign, Illinois.

Anxiety, Panic Attacks, and MVPS

Research studies confirm that many MVPers do have anxiety and panic attacks. The connection between the two, however, remains unclear. A heightened autonomic nervous system may be partly responsible.

Before you begin this chapter, see how much you already know. Take the following quiz. Check either true or false.

QUIZ

1. To feel anxiety means I fail to cope.
   True _____ False _____

2. If my heart palpitates and my hands tingle,
   a fatal heart attack follows.
   True _____ False _____

3. Panic attacks come out of the blue.
   True _____ False _____

4. I can do nothing about panic attacks.
   True _____ False _____

All of the above statements are false. Now, read on.

Remember, there's *no cure* for MVP, but you *can learn* to peacefully co-exist with it. Don't turn over your life to chronic heath conditions such as: MVPS, arthritis, hypertension, or diabetes. If you do, expect to feel like a *cork bobbing in the ocean* always waiting for the next big wave, shark, or typhoon. A helpless, out-of-control feeling leads to depression, anxiety, phobias, or panic attacks. Right now make it a goal to take charge of your life. How?

Become knowledgeable. Knowledge *is* power. Carefully read, reread, and *study* this chapter because panic attacks *don't come out of the blue*. How then, might *you* trigger these attacks? How can you avoid them?

Anxiety

Webster defines anxiety as a state of being uneasy, apprehensive, or worried about what *might* happen — a concern about some *possible* future event. Anxiety is a normal living experience: physically, emotionally, socially, spiritually, and psychologically.

The word anxiety is sometimes misconstrued. Anxiety, for example, is the psychological siren of the human organism. Remember your first date, your wedding day, the birth of your first child? How did you feel? Did your heart pound? Were you faint, dizzy, or weak? Would it be fair to say that you felt anxious? Yes, of course.

Throughout life, anxiety normally occurs at various developmental transition points. Children learn to crawl and walk because they're frustrated *and* anxious. They want the shiny red ball across the room. As their hearts pound, and their limbs tremble, they move under their own power for the first time. Thus, they overcome their anxiety and grow. In moderation, anxiety encourages growth. In excess, anxiety paralyzes and sometimes causes panic attacks.

What produces anxiety in one person doesn't necessarily produce anxiety in another. For example: Some people fear flying. Others fear driving. Some fear open spaces. Others fear confined areas.

Research demonstrates that anxiety and panic are controlled and governed by an individual's *perception*. How you perceive something influences your emotions the way you think and the way you feel. If you perceive MVPS symptoms as catastrophic, you *encourage* a panic attack. Alter your *perception*, and you control it. *You* are the only one who is in charge of your panic attacks.

Anatomy of Panic Attacks

What kinds of feelings characterize panic attacks?

In the absence of any *external* threats, brief episodes of intense fear occur and surface as physical symptoms. They often inflict terror and a fear of losing control. Symptoms may last several seconds or for several minutes. Anyone who has experienced an attack characterizes it as frightening and most uncomfortable. In fact, you sometimes momentarily think, "I'm losing my mind."

Panic attacks resemble fight-or-flight responses. For example: Suppose you walk in Central Park in New York at midnight and suddenly hear a strange sound. Bursts of catecholamines — adrenaline-like substances — activate and circulate throughout your system. Now, you shake; you perspire. Your heart pounds; your muscles tense; your breathing accelerates. You prepare to flee or to fight.

In much the same way, this area of the brain that controls the fight-or-flight response stimulates and sets off panic attacks. But, now this alarm — this danger response — occurs *even though there's no real danger.*

A panic attack often occurs following any form of severe stress Examples: divorce, illness, job change, work overload, serious accident, or loss of a family member. (Also, excessive consumption of caffeine, or use of stimulant medications may trigger panic attacks.)

With recurring panic attacks, it is not uncommon for you to *anticipate* another attack. This behavior — fear of having another panic attack — is called *anticipatory anxiety.* Afflicted persons become apprehensive and often begin to avoid any events and circumstances likely to trigger attacks. For example, if you had your first or worst anxiety attack while driving, anticipatory anxiety may keep you from driving again. As more attacks occur in different settings, the person's activities may become increasingly limited. Family, social, and professional activities become severely disrupted. The person may become agoraphobic.[1]

Agoraphobia affects approximately one-third of all people with panic disorder. They fear being in any place or situation where escape might be difficult, or where help is unavailable in the event of a panic attack. Commonly, people with agoraphobia fear crowds, standing in line, entering shopping malls, and riding in cars or in public transportation. Often, their comfort zone includes only their home or immediate neighborhood. At times, they may travel if accompanied by a friend. Even when they are in their comfort zone, they may continue to have panic attacks.

---

[1]Agora is Greek for marketplace. Agoraphobia literally means fear of the marketplace — a fear of crowds of people assembled there.

PANIC ATTACK SYMPTOMS

During a panic attack, any or all of the following symptoms occur:

- Terror — a sense that something horrible is about to happen and you're powerless to prevent it

- Shortness of breath

- Smothering sensation

- Dizziness, unsteady feelings, or faintness

- Palpitations or tachycardia — rapid heart rate

- Trembling or shaking

- Sweating

- Choking — numbness or tingling sensations

- Nausea or abdominal distress

- Flushes — hot flashes — or chills

- Chest pain or discomfort

- Fear of dying

- Fear of going crazy or of doing something uncontrolled

Source: National Institute of Mental Health, 1993

Perceptions

Research indicates that panic attacks result from the catastrophic misinterpretation of certain bodily sensations. This is illustrated below.

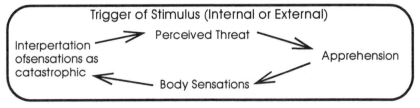

Source: Clark, D. (1986).

"OUT OF THE BLUE?"

An exchange between an MVP program participant, Laura, and the seminar leader follows.

Laura: "My last panic attack occurred at home as I sat at my computer. Nothing happened to cause it. The attack literally came out of the blue. What do you mean it didn't?"

Seminar leader: "Let's explore the time period before the attack."

Laura: "It wasn't a good week. My husband was out of town. I always get edgy when he's away. *I'm afraid something will happen.* It never has; but, it could. I'm responsible for three little children — you never know what can happen."

She further recalled, "I ate a large meal before I began to work. Eating a full meal frequently causes palpitations. I remember I had palpitations when I first began to work at my computer."

Now, Laura began to place the panic attack into its proper context. As she explored the time period immediately *before* the attack, she realized her palpitations were more intense than usual. She believed she was going to die. As the palpitations intensified, she became even more anxious than usual.

Because the physical symptom is perceived as very intense, there's an increased risk to misinterpret it as catastrophic. When Laura put the situation into perspective, it became apparent that her physical symptom — palpitations — became catastrophically misinterpreted. Faced with a perceived threat, she had no choice but to have a panic attack.

To apply this illustration, think of *internal trigger stimuli* as palpitations, dizziness, or chest pain, and of *external stimuli* as flying, driving, shopping in supermarkets. Any stimulus perceived as a threat causes you to become apprehensive. For example, you may say, "I hope I don't have a panic attack while I'm driving." Soon, your heart pounds; your chest hurts; and you become short of breath. Each bodily sensation intensifies with apprehension. Each sensation becomes catastrophic. You're convinced that because you have a heart problem and chest pains, you're going to die.

In Chapter 1 you learned that your autonomic nervous system automatically becomes stimulated by *perceived* threats. Your body normally responds and causes you to perspire, to feel breathless and dizzy, or to note pounding heartbeats. If these normal physical responses are misinterpreted as catastrophic, the panic cycle feeds on itself and perpetuates.

To say panic attacks occur *out of the blue*, contradicts findings gained through research. Studies show that *panic attacks are triggered by a physical sensation* such as palpitations. In turn, the physical sensation increases both awareness and an anxiety level that intensifies the physical responses of the autonomic nervous system. This is interpreted as catastrophic, and the threat is intensified. Finally, anxiety escalates to panic level and sends the autonomic nervous system into overdrive. To try and stop a panic attack at this point is similar to putting your car in reverse while driving 70 miles an hour.

As you saw, the time and place to act on an impending attack is *before* it happens — *before* you interpret harmless, normal physical signs — palpitations, tingling, dizziness — as *catastrophic*. Prevent your autonomic nervous system from going into overdrive.

If you don't like *how* you feel about yourself, about your life, and about your symptoms, *change* how you *think*. It's the key to taking control of anxiety and panic attacks. How? Try cognitive therapy.

Cognitive Therapy

Cognition includes all forms of knowing: perceiving, judging, conceiving, reasoning, and remembering. According to cognitive therapy, abnormalities of behavior and mood result from abnormal thinking. Cognitive therapy, therefore, gives priority to thinking and not to feelings. It is a helpful tool to use on your own.

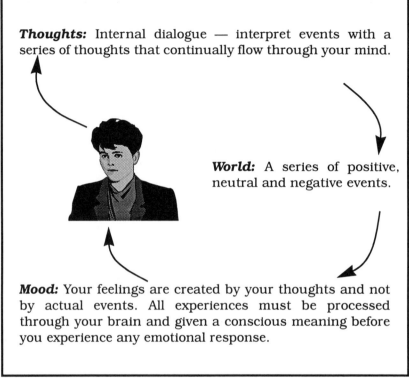

Thoughts: Internal dialogue — interpret events with a series of thoughts that continually flow through your mind.

World: A series of positive, neutral and negative events.

Mood: Your feelings are created by your thoughts and not by actual events. All experiences must be processed through your brain and given a conscious meaning before you experience any emotional response.

Source: Burns, D. (1980).

Guiding Principles of Cognitive Therapy

Principle 1 — Automatic Thoughts: Moods and feelings are influenced in the here-and-now by automatic thoughts and cognitions. These automatic thoughts create a stream of ideas that repeatedly and insistently intrude upon our conscious awareness.

Examples of problematic automatic thoughts associated with MVPS: "I have MVPS; something is wrong with my heart. If my heart goes, my body follows." Whenever this MVPer has palpitations his thought process *will* interpret palpitations as catastrophic.

Principle 2 — Thought Traps or Cognitive Distortions: Pessimistic thoughts that cause depression and anxiety frequently are unrealistic, illogical, and distorted. A common denominator in thought distortions is *negativity*. When nothing is good and nowhere is safe, chronic depression and high-level anxiety ensue. *Reality doesn't cause* unhealthy feelings such as depression or anxiety. Rather, negative thoughts about reality contribute.

Ten forms of cognitive distortions, or twisted thinking, that create negative emotions include:[2]

1. All-or-Nothing Thinking: You see everything as black and white with no gray areas. You're a total failure if one aspect of your life is less than perfect. For example, if your boss makes a minor correction on your report, you know he will fire you. You're incompetent.

2. Overgeneralization: You set up a self-fulfilling prophecy of defeat based on one negative event. Examples: The alarm failed to go off this morning. You're sure the car won't start. You'll be late for work. Your boss will hate your presentation. By tomorrow morning, you'll be a bag lady.

3. Mental Filter: You focus on a single negative detail and create a dark reality. Example: After you receive many compliments on your presentation, someone recommends using blue instead of black ink. You leave the meeting depressed.

4. Discounting the Positive: You insist your positive qualities or accomplishments don't count. Example: Your sister says you look like a knockout in your dress. You politely tell her what she says doesn't count — she's family.

5. Jumping to Conclusions: In the absence of accurate information, you believe the worst.

(a) *Mind reading:* Everyone dislikes you.

(b) *Fortune-telling:* You predict that everything will turn out badly.

Example: Although your friend was on the second level of the mall and you were on the first, surely she intentionally ignored you. She didn't wave hello. She will never talk to you again.

6. Catastrophizing or Minimizing: You discount the positive and accentuate the negative. Example: Because your friend complains for hours about how she had to change part of her

---

[2]Burns, D. 1980. Feeling Good: The New Mood Therapy; Burns, D. 1993. Ten Days to Self Esteem.

presentation, you empathize. Even though the company accepted *your* proposal you say how *bad* it is.

7. *Emotional Reasoning:*   You believe that your worst fears and feelings are reality. Example: You receive a call. The boss wants to see you. Since this only could mean he wants to fire you, you suffer a panic attack on the elevator enroute to his office.

8. *"Should" Statements:*   You criticize yourself or others with *shoulds*.

Shoulds usually indicate two seemingly conflicting sets of needs. Failure to choose between the two and accept the consequences, causes discomfort. Example: I should visit my parents every week. Mothers should meet all the needs of all members of their family. Men should never show weakness. I should never feel anxious. I should never get angry. I should never have palpitations if my heart is truly OK.

9. *Labeling:*   You make yourself the sum total of what you do; you attach value to yourself *based only on what you do*. Example: Instead of saying, "I forgot to make the appointment — I made a mistake," you tell yourself, "I'm a loser — I can't do anything right."

10. *Personalization:*   You see yourself as the *cause* of every negative event with which you come in contact. Example: Your husband is angry and short with you. You know *you* caused it.

As you see, to feel *bad* about yourself comes from distorted thought patterns. Distorted thoughts won't let you feel *good* about yourself. What can you do? Replace negative, unrealistic thoughts with positive, realistic thoughts. Yes, you *can* change the way you feel.

Positive reinforcement and good feelings about yourself are the sustenance that feed a stable and secure sense of self. MVPers who possess a stable and secure self usually operate at a relatively low anxiety level. Furthermore, the less daily anxiety you experience, the less likely you perceive MVPS symptoms as life threatening and panic.

Principle 3 — Believing in Incorrect Assumptions about Oneself and One's Self-esteem: Attaching your self-esteem, or sense of well-being to the success of a project, to the response from another, or to the presence or absence of a mistake, makes feeling good impossible. Faulty assumptions cause fear, anxiety, and panic.

Examples of faulty assumptions: Because you haven't had palpitations in a week, you'll never have them again. If MVPS is harmless, you should never have any symptoms. Believe your worth as a human being depends on what you do.

In each of these situations, you assume a cause-and-effect relationship between nonrelated items. Example: MVPS is not curable. Expect occasional symptoms. Don't base your sense of well-being on never having any symptoms. You'll set yourself up for anxiety and panic attacks.

Furthermore, the belief that self-worth depends on one's achievements leads to a roller-coaster ride through life. One's self-worth and self-esteem come from inside. You'll note that it is called *self*-esteem, and not *the-other-person-gives-it-to-you* esteem. It's a constant sense of knowing who you are, why you are the way you are, and what you believe you're capable of doing in any situation. If you're only as good as your project, you hand over responsibility for how you feel about yourself to other people, i.e., to a committee, or to anyone who approves your project. These people don't take responsibility for *your* self-esteem. Instead, they concern themselves with only *their own* self-esteem. Therefore, only *you* can assume responsibility and determine how you feel about yourself.

Although feedback is important, place it in the context of your entire social, physical, spiritual, psychological, and intellectual being. You *are* more than the sum of all the tasks you've done. To believe otherwise leads to chronic anxiety. Then, everything you do has the potential to make you feel terrible about yourself. How much of that can any one person take without becoming anxious, depressed, and panicky?

Goals of Cognitive Therapy

To take control, strive to achieve the following goals:

1. Pinpoint automatic thoughts, thought traps, and silent assumptions that trigger and perpetuate anxiety or panic-attack cycles.

2. Identify the distortions or cognitive errors.

3. Substitute more realistic, self-enhancing thoughts that reduce painful feelings.

4. Replace self-defeating, silent assumptions with more reasonable-belief systems.

If you now believe: My heart pounds; I have chest pain; I have MVPS; I'm having a heart attack, change your thinking. Say to yourself, "I've had this before; this is not new to me. I didn't die before, and I'm *not* going to die now."

Continue to perceive your palpitations as catastrophic, and you choose to have a panic attack. Don't perceive them as catastrophic, and choose to avert an attack. Remember, *you* can recreate the perception you created.

Start your own personal cognitive therapy now. Think about your last attack. What happened in your life the day before, the hour before the attack? Complete the *Thought Analysis Sheet* (Burns, 1993). Fill in the spaces in whatever order you remember.

At the top of the sheet, briefly describe the situation that led to your physical response. In the first column, list any physical symptoms you felt: palpitations, chest pain, numbness, or shortness of breath. Next, record your emotional response and any cognitive distortion. In the last column, write a rational response to your thoughts.

The critical step is the positive or rational response. *Be open and honest with yourself.* Thus, you'll begin: to challenge your automatic thoughts, to identify your thought traps, and to discover your anxiety producing assumptions. Be surprised by the results; but, remember this is a process.

Start with hindsight, and realize you lost control just *after the attack*. Now, realize what you did *while it went on* but couldn't stop it. This helps you identify situations that place you at risk of an attack. Examples: flying, driving, eating, being alone, or during the middle of the night. Although you may still have another attack, you'll know what's happening to you. As you continue to use this process, you'll feel symptoms: tingling, palpitations, chest pain, feelings of unreality, but you'll recognize them. Although you're scared, you'll know they are normal, but not fatal.

Remember, **ANXIETY IS NOT TERMINAL**. Anxiety, and its physical manifestations, are normal occurrences. Catastrophic misinterpretations of the body's *normal* response to *normal* anxiety cause panic attacks. Although cognitive therapy is *not* a substitute for medicine or for psychotherapy, it is a useful tool. It provides a structure for altering the incidence of panic attacks. Start now. Use the work sheet. Soon you'll be able to mentally complete the sheet.

Examples:

Situation: *I have to drive to the supermarket where I had my first anxiety attack.*

THOUGHT ANALYSIS SHEET

PHYSICAL SYMPTOM	COGNITIVE DISTORTION	POSITIVE THOUGHT
Heart pounding	I'm going to die (Emotional reasoning)	I've had heart pounding before. I can do pursed-lip breathing and feel better.

Situation: *My husband is out of town. I worry that something might happen to me and my children will be alone.*

THOUGHT ANALYSIS SHEET

PHYSICAL SYMPTOM	COGNITIVE DISTORTION	POSITIVE THOUGHT
Chest pain	I'm going to have a heart attack. (Catastrophizing) (Emotional reasoning)	Nothing has ever happened that I couldn't handle when he was out of town. I don't like being alone, but I can manage. Actually, chest pains are part of MVPS, and my fear makes them worse.

Situation: *The boss wants to see me now. I decide to take the stairs to his office.*

THOUGHT ANALYSIS SHEET

PHYSICAL SYMPTOM	COGNITIVE DISTORTION	POSITIVE THOUGHT
Short of breath Dizziness Heart pounding	I'm going to be fired. He hates me. My heartbeat is going to kill me. (Emotional reasoning) (Catastrophizing) (Emotional reasoning)	I don't know what the boss wants. My fear makes my MVPS symptoms worse. If I breathe deeply and slow my pace down, I'll be fine.

Situation: _____

THOUGHT ANALYSIS SHEET

PHYSICAL SYMPTOM	COGNITIVE DISTORTION	POSITIVE THOUGHT

Medications

For completeness, medications often prescribed for the treatment of panic attacks are discussed below. The intent of this section is to provide information, *not* to recommend one drug over another, nor suggest you start taking medication. For many, symptoms are managed without medication. Some people, however, may temporarily need or want medication to get over the hump. Together with your physician discuss the use of medication, its purpose, its effectiveness, and its accompanying guidelines.

Commonly used medications to treat panic attacks include antidepressants and anti-anxiety agents — minor tranquilizers. Some forms of depression have a *major anxiety component* that can induce anxiety symptoms. Therefore, to medically treat the depression can decrease anxiety and the risk of panic attacks. The pharmacological actions of the drugs are complex, and beyond the scope of this chapter.

Tofranil — Imipramine — is a tricyclic antidepressant (TCA) frequently used in the treatment of panic attacks. Common side effects include dry mouth and constipation. To alleviate dry mouth, chew sugar-free gum or hard candy. To minimize constipation, increase your water intake to at least eight glasses per day. If water doesn't help, drink prune juice or use a mild laxative. Notify your physician should you experience sweating, extreme nervousness, blurred vision, or flushing of the face.

Recently, a newer classification of antidepressants the SSRI's — Serotonin Specific Re-uptake Inhibitors are used to treat anxiety and panic conditions. Examples of these medications include Zoloft and Paxil. The popularity of these medications can be attributed to their effectiveness, and fewer side effects than tricyclic antidepressants. They work by affecting Serotonin a naturally occurring neurotransmitter that functions as the body's calmative substance. Medications such as Zoloft and Paxil increase the availability of serotonin in the body, and thereby help prevent panic attacks.

A group of antidepressants known as MAO inhibitors are also used to treat panic attacks. Examples: Nardil — Phenelzine — and Parnate — tranylcypromine. Side effects include sleep disturbance, weight gain, and sexual dysfunction. When you take MAO inhibitors, *closely monitor your diet*. Foods that contain high amounts of tyramine can interact with MAO inhibitors and cause serious side effects such as a sharp, dangerous rise in blood pressure.

FOODS TO AVOID WITH MAO INHIBITORS
- Beer and wine, particularly Chianti
- Cheese, except cottage and cream cheese
- Smoked or pickled fish, especially herring
- Beef or chicken liver
- Summer sausage — dry
- Fava or broad bean pods — Italian green beans
- Yeast vitamin supplements — brewer's yeast
- Ripe fresh banana
- Ripe avocado
- Sour cream
- Soy sauce
- Yogurt
- Yeast breads
- Raisins
- Figs
- Meat tenderizers
- Chocolate
- Caffeine-containing beverages

A twenty-eight-year-old woman cancelled two appointments with the MVP Program. Each time, enroute to the center, she suffered panic attacks. The third time her husband drove, and she had no problem.

It was three months after her daughter's birth, that panic attacks began. She endured a difficult pregnancy, was on bed rest the last three months and then delivered a baby who became colicky. Needless to say, the new mother's panic attacks increased in intensity and in frequency. Furthermore, with the husband's transfer, they now lived in a city 200 miles from the only home she ever knew.

At The MVP Program, we began with a family history. Although she knew little about MVPS, she remembered her father's taking medication for nerves. Her sister, an aerobics instructor, seemed to be high strung but kept it under control with exercise. She then asked if a lack of exercise may have played a role in *her* own panic attacks. Ever since high school and until pregnancy, she ran 25 miles a week.

I said, "YES. Exercise produces endorphins that are involved in the synthesis of serotonin. Serotonin is the neurotransmitter involved in mental alertness and systemic calming. Through exercise you previously compensated for an apparent familial chemical imbalance."

Together, we developed a plan that involved diet, exercise, and thought analysis. She agreed to follow the plan for three months. *Unless* she experienced a decrease in frequency and intensity of her panic attacks, she would return. Only then would we discuss medication to help her bring a degree of control and mastery into her life. For two years now, I have not seen her.

In addition to dietary recommendations, avoid over-the-counter medications that contain vasopressor substances — ephedrine or phenylpropanolamine. Examples include: Contact and Dristan. Be certain your physician gives you information about any dietary and medication restrictions.

Antidepressants take at least 14 days to reach full effect. When you become stabilized at a dose, you should notice a decrease in the frequency of panic attacks. It may take several months; so don't stop the medicine because you feel better and haven't had a panic attack. Your body needs to finally take over and do what the medicine did. Work with your physician to gradually decrease the medicine over a period of time. If panic attacks return during withdrawal, one of two things might be happening. First, you may have a chemical imbalance. This may require continued treatment with medication. Second, perhaps you depended solely upon the medicine and did little to help yourself.

Minor tranquilizers or anti-anxiety agents such as Xanax — alprazolam — and Ativan — lorezepam — are used either to stop or prevent an attack when conditions seem conducive. These agents relax you and help you to think better. Less anxious, you'll be less inclined to catastrophically interpret something. If you're in the throes of an attack, Xanax may help blunt the symptoms.

Anti-anxiety agents are addictive, and in time you'll require higher doses to do the job. If you took several a day and *every day* for many months, work with your physician to gradually decrease the dosage and discontinue the medication. Remember, medication *does not cure* the problem. You must continue to work at helping yourself.

Frequently Asked Questions about Anxiety and Panic Attacks

1. I've had MVP for years, and panic attacks that start and stop. How come?

Panic attacks often come and go during changes in your life. Here is one theory.

In the growing fetus, the nervous system and the heart develop simultaneously. If one develops defectively, so may the other. The result might be but a *hair trigger* on your fight-or-flight response.

Compared with most people, an MVPer's autonomic nervous system can respond quicker, and with greater intensity. When this sensitive nervous system is subjected to a series of stressors that occur within a short period of time, a panic attack can occur. This is called the *kindling effect*. The faulty nervous system may predispose you to the development of symptoms. With the right amount of stressors, in the right amount of time, a panic attack ensues. You may , however, never develop symptoms till your life situation challenges.

Stressors are *kindling* for the development of panic attacks. For example: Are you starting a new job, moving away from home, getting a divorce, fighting with your neighbors, raising a family, and working full time? These are typical major stressors that can cause panic. But it doesn't need to be a major stressor. Instead, an assortment of minor stressors may cause panic attacks. Examples: The kids are sick. The baby sitter quit. Your car broke down, and your mother wants to go shopping today. Whatever raises your daily anxiety level beyond baseline, increases your risk of having a panic attack, as well as increasing the intensity and frequency of MVPS symptoms. The cycle goes on.

2. What is the difference between an anxiety state and a panic attack?

Anxiety is normal; a panic attack paralyzes. Anxiety means perceiving something as threatening. Example: taking a driver's test. If you're having a panic attack, you've perceived something as catastrophic. I'm going to accidently run over the driving inspector.

3. What do I do when I'm having an attack? How do I cope with a panic attack?

When you have a panic attack, the goal is to keep safe while you ride it out. In its early stages, walk around and concentrate on deep breathing. This may blunt or calm symptoms. Physical activity gives panic impulses along your nervous system some competition. If you have someone you can talk to, call that person. If a tranquilizer has been prescribed for you, take it. The medicine helps you to relax and lessen the intensity of your symptoms. As you relax and consider these symptoms to be normal, your autonomic nervous system switches from fight-or-flight to a steady, controlled state.

If all attempts fail and you seriously feel that you are going to die, go to an emergency room. You and your well-being are worth it.

Remember, the time to act on a panic attack is *before* it happens. Stopping a Ferrari at full throttle is difficult. As soon as possible after a panic attack use the Thought-Analysis Sheet. Identify which perceptions induced an attack. Replace misinformation with correct information. You control your perceptions. You control panic attacks.

4. Is it possible to awaken at night with an anxiety attack?

Yes. Through dreams we take care of any issues, concerns, and feelings that we failed to address during the day. Combined with even low levels of stressful, depressing, and anxiety producing events, a panic attack can occur during sleep. Thus, when we fail to remember the dream that perhaps precipitated an attack, we entertain weird thoughts. For example: "I must be dying because I can't find any reason *why* I'm having a panic attack." Then, when sleep becomes a problem, the baseline-anxiety level escalates. Hence, the cycle intensifies and perpetuates.

As one approach to solving this problem, place a pen and a note pad beside your bed. Say to yourself before retiring, "I *will* remember my dreams tonight." As soon as you awaken, write *whatever* you remember about the dream. From these bits and pieces plus an analysis of you presleep anxiety level, you may learn what caused a panic attack.

5. Is anger related to panic attacks?

Yes. If you are angry, your life may not be going the way you wish. That spells stress. Stress can be acted out or expressed through a weakened body part. Examples: Migraines, ulcers, colitis, spastic colon, and back pain. MVPS symptoms sometimes act out stress in a similar fashion. Anger and associated stress can cause an increase in the severity and frequency of symptoms such as palpitations and chest pain. The more intense the symptom pattern, greater is the likelihood of a catastrophic interpretation and risk of a panic attack. Yes, panic attacks and anger are closely related.

6. Does cognitive therapy really work?

Yes, it does. Cognitive therapy gets you off *automatic pilot* responding to the symptoms of the panic attack as if you're only along for the ride. Cognitive therapy prepares you to become your own master. You recognize symptoms that evoke panic attacks, learn how to control them, and, in turn, learn how to prevent them in the future.

Said one MVPer. "I really let this thing get the best of me. I couldn't even go to the grocery store for fear I'd have a panic attack. Now, I *don't think* I'm about to die with palpitations. Instead, I talk to them and say, 'I know you're there; but, I'm busy. Now, let's get it over.' People think I'm crazy, but this works well for me."

7. Are there any other ways to cope with anxiety and panic attacks in addition to using cognitive therapy?

Yes. Learn ways to relax and to keep your anxiety level below threshold. Participate in a cardiovascular exercise program. Exercise helps *siphon off any charge*. Once anxiety approaches a livable level, you're more inclined to risk uncovering your sources of anxiety.

Relaxation provides a key to self mastery. As you work off frustrations and insecurities through exercise, you put yourself in a positive frame of mind, prepared to uncover and to treat any *sources* of anxiety. Consult a trained therapist to learn about biofeedback through the use of relaxation tapes.

Become knowledgeable about diet. For example, did you know that carbohydrates play a major role in either preventing or decreasing the intensity of panic attacks? Processing of carbohydrates in the body boosts the availability of tryptophan. Tryptophan — an amino acid involved in the synthesis of serotonin — is the neurotransmitter that helps us control mood, feel calm, concentrated, focused, relaxed, and content.

Unfortunately, because we often eat carbohydrates with protein or fat we *decrease* the availability of tryptophan.

Carbohydrates are an effective anxiety reducing agent when eaten alone. Recommended servings include: 2 oz. of oyster crackers, 16 animal crackers, 1 plain bagel, 2.5 oz. of pretzels, and 1-1/2 cups of Alpha Bits. Allow 30 minutes to work. Eaten in moderation prior to a high-risk event (driving a car, going to the supermarket, a visit from your mother-in-law), carbohydrates can be an effective, nonpharmaceutical, chemical intervention to reduce anxiety. This intervention is within *your control*, no prescription, no authorization needed.

Remember to avoid foods that create stress. These include: caffeine, fried foods, junk foods, and sugar. Also, if you enjoy herbal teas, try catnip, hops, passion flower, chamomile, and valerian root. These have a calming effect.

8. When should I seek help from a therapist?

If, after three months of regular exercise, a modified diet, and use of thought-analysis sheets, there is no decrease in either the frequency or intensity of your panic attacks, its time to seek help. Something else is happening. Unless effectively treated, depression, chemical imbalance, or both cause symptoms to persist.

Interview prospective therapists, as you would new employees. Learn what they know about MVPS Do they use the cognitive approach in the treatment of panic attacks? What is their position on the use of medication to bring panic attacks under control? Then, choose a therapist with an advanced degree — master's or doctorate — who is associated with a physician. This therapist can work with you on two levels.

On level one, is the use of medication to stabilize your nervous system. Because medication is self administered, it helps you build a sense of mastery over the panic attacks.

On level two, both you and the therapist address the possible *source* of your depression. Once identified, together, you lay the groundwork for the next step — prevention. Say to yourself, "Although I am responsible for my depression, I also have the willpower to *get* myself out and the willpower to keep myself out." In therapy, *knowledge is power*. Make sure that the therapist you choose agrees.

9. My sister and I both have MVPS. I have panic attacks. She doesn't. Why?

Not every person with MVPS even knows that he or she has it. Furthermore, *not everyone* with MVPS has panic attacks. The best explanation of these realities lies in the examination of one's "internal climate."

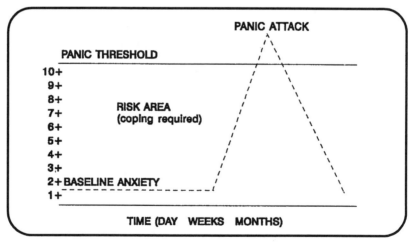

Everyone operates with a degree of anxiety known as a *base-line*-anxiety level. (See diagram). Each person has a panic threshold: the amount of anxiety generated to cause a panic attack. Our baseline-anxiety level fluctuates according to how well we manage ourselves, and how we perceive stresses that come our way. Given enough stressors over a short period of time together with poor stress management such as thought traps and automatic thoughts, we *can* reach the panic level, and a panic attack ensues.

10. How do I deal with friends and family?

The answer is twofold: accept responsibility for the manner in which you *react* to MVPS; *within reason* enlighten friends and family members concerning its symptoms. Explain how they come and go, and why they sometimes become problematical.

Too, no one but *you* can improve your condition. Parents, spouses, children, and friends do *not* have the responsibility to make your condition better. To expect others' lives to revolve around *you* invites rejection. If you believe, "If only they would do, say, or be ... I wouldn't have panic attacks," you may feel unloved, depressed, and anxious. Your relationships will be fraught with conflict, blame, and distance. The result is more MVPS symptoms.

To expect others to shoulder responsibility they're unable to do, keeps you from gaining mastery over a condition that is *your* responsibility. Once you accept the responsibility for your panic attacks, you allow family and friends to fulfill their role as a support system. They too need information to understand changes you make in relationships. Although friends and family may not appreciate limit setting and boundary changes, given the proper information, they may be more tolerant. Keep in mind that it's never easy to accept whatever we don't understand.

Summary

You are not alone. Many other MVPers suffer from anxiety and panic attacks. From this book you know that anxiety is a normal human response to a perceived threat. Also, that a panic attack starts when a normal physical reaction to a perceived threat is catastrophically interpreted. Keep in mind that *you are in control* of what is perceived as a threat.

Use cognitive therapy as a tool for you to identify any perceptions, faulty assumptions, and thought distortions that contribute to the intensity and frequency of your panic attacks.

Next, *correct* your faulty assumptions, and get rid of all perceptual and thought distortions. Be determined; begin right now. *Take control* over your anxiety and panic attacks. And, don't forget: What you think determines how you feel. To like the way you feel, change the way you think. *The choice is YOURS.*

References

Balch, J., & Balch, P. 1990. *Prescription for Nutritional Healing.* Avery Publishing Group Inc. Garden City Park, New York.

Burns, D. 1980. *Feeling good: The New Mood Therapy.* William Morrow and Company, Inc. New York.

Burns, D. 1989. *The Feeling Good Handbook.* William Morrow and Company, Inc. New York.

Burns, D. 1993. *Ten Days to Self-esteem: The Leader's Manual.* William Morrow and Company, Inc. New York.

Childress, A., & Burns, D. 1981. "The basics of cognitive therapy." *Psychosomatics.* **12**: 1017–1027.

Clark, D. 1986. "A cognitive approach to panic." *Behavior Research and Therapy.* **4**: 461–470.

Amsterdam, E., Carter, C., Holloway, R., & Schwenk, T. 1994. "Is it normal worry — or pathologic anxiety?" *Patient Care.* 26–29.

Gelder, M. 1983. "Is cognitive therapy effective?" Discussion paper. *Journal of the Royal Society of Medicine.* **11**: 938–942.

National Institute of Mental Health. "Panic Disorder in the Medical Setting," by Katon, W. NIH Publication No. 93-3482. Washington, DC: Supt. of Docs., U.S. Govt. Print Off., 1993.

Rapp, M. (1980). "Cognitive therapy: An early appraisal." *Canadian Journal of Psychiatry.* **25**: 332–337.

Starting a Support Group

"Living with MVPS isn't easy. I wish I had others to talk to who understand. Is there a support group in my area?"

"I want to start a support group. How do I begin? Can you help?"

Callers to The MVP Program of Cincinnati repeatedly ask these questions. As you note at the end of this chapter, although thousands suffer with MVPS, few support groups exist.

What is a Support Group?

It is a self-help group that brings together individuals with common goals and concerns. Within the group, members learn they're not alone — their fears, feelings, and hopes aren't the-exception, they're the rule. Meeting together encourages problem solving by an individual or by a group. When people share, they learn from one another. They gain new insights, become more-confident, and enjoy a feeling of accomplishment.

Led by and for their members, these groups are also described as mutual-help groups, and hundreds already exist for a variety of reasons. Keep in mind that it took people with a little bit of courage, a sense of commitment, and a lot of caring to start each group. Examples: Alcoholic-Anonymous, Mended Hearts, and Parents without Partners.

A support group need not meet indefinitely. For example, you may meet a specific goal within a short period of time. On the other hand, a support group may continue for years with different members entering and leaving as their needs change.

Never lose sight, however, because no support group can meet *all the needs, wants, and desires of all of its members all of the time*. Furthermore, MVP self-help groups certainly are not designed to be psychotherapy groups. Groups with a psychotherapy focus require professional leaders with special training.

How Does Someone Start a Support Group?

Who starts an MVP support group? YOU do. If you were not born a support-group leader, you *can* become one. Furthermore, you need not reinvent the wheel. Instead, learn from others who have done it before. Many cities have health-related, self-help support groups. To locate them, check with your local self-help clearinghouse or the help lines serving your area. Review community papers for time, date, and place of support-group meetings. Attend meetings, and speak with the leaders. If you're unable to find a local group, call an MVP support group listed at the end of the chapter.

Benefit from the group's successes and failures. By doing so, gain confidence, and decide to start a support group. Write for starter packets or any other helpful materials. Be sure to enclose a large, self-addressed and adequately stamped envelope. Many groups work on a tight budget.

Spread the word in your community. How? Contact church groups, civic groups, and school administrators. Post fliers in busy places such as: grocery stores, libraries, beauty shops, barber shops, bingo halls. Don't worry about reaching people without MVPS — they may have friends who are looking for a group like yours. Fliers need to simply state, "Looking for energetic people to help start a support group for those with Mitral Valve Prolapse Syndrome. Call (give phone number) between (give time) 5:00 P.M. and 9:00 P.M."

In response to calls, clearly state your expectations. Ask callers if they agree to participate in discussions and share their experiences with MVPS. Will they also involve themselves and help on committees? Some people enthusiastically volunteer to help start a support group and share responsibilities. Others wait for someone else to take over. Don't despair.

Instead, seek help from friends or from health-care professionals sensitive to your needs. For example, contact nurses in cardiologists' offices. If unable to participate, they may refer you to someone else who is knowledgeable and available.

Call the editor of your local newspaper. Ask whether or not he publishes announcements of meetings within the community and without charge. If so, say you're interested because you are starting an MVPS-support group in the area.

To spark his interest and to possibly get a feature story published, *briefly* explain that MVPS sometimes mimics a full-blown heart attack; it is sometimes misdiagnosed; and it is often a traumatic experience. Invite a reporter to attend a meeting, and offer to loan him this book for additional information.

Provided you do publish notices of meetings, keep them simple. Example: "Please attend a support-group meeting for people with Mitral Valve Prolapse Syndrome. **Date, Time**, **Specific place, and Address. Phone (give number)** from 5:00 P.M. to 9:00 P.M. **(give appropriate time when someone will be available).**

Example of a printed flier:

DO YOU, TOO, SUFFER WITH MITRAL VALVE PROLAPSE SYNDROME? JOIN OTHERS AT A FIRST SUPPORT-GROUP MEETING.

DATE: May 8th

TIME: 6:00 P.M.

LOCATION: Mighty Valuable Players' House
The Tor Room
1968 Taconic Road
River Park, NY 12345

For further information call Lisa at (012) 232-4573 before 8:00 P.M.

Carefully read this chapter for suggestions; but, use it as only a guide about group dynamics, leadership, problem solving, and more — see references at the end of the chapter.

How Do I Organize and Conduct the First Meeting?

Choose a date and time — preferably evening — that doesn't pose a serious conflict. Review community, school, college, and professional sports calendars. Check newspapers for local events. Even an eager person may find it difficult to attend a meeting during final exams or on baseball's opening day. Later on, should members prefer to change the dates and time of meetings, follow-the wishes of the majority.

Select a meeting place in a convenient location — preferably a place that's free of charge. As a suggestion — inquire at a mall, school, church, synagogue, YMCA, or YWCA, hospital, university, library, or community center. If you anticipate a small group, have the first meeting in someone's home. Be certain the meeting place is easily accessible, and its location promotes a sense of security or well being.

As a group leader, arrive ahead of time. Place chairs in a circle, *without* a special chair for the leader.

Be a good hostess. As people arrive, make them feel welcome. Provide blank stick-on tags and a dry-mark pen for name tags. Direct them to refreshments and to the meeting area. Also, indicate where rest rooms are located. Keep an attendance book with names, addresses, and telephone numbers. Ask each attendant to regularly sign in.

To begin the meeting, introduce yourself. Then say, "Take a partner — not your spouse or your good friend — but someone you don't already know. Interview each other during the next five minutes and get acquainted." Then, ask partners around the circle to introduce *each other*. As each one acknowledges the introduction, ask her to briefly tell something about herself. Allow one or two minutes for each introduction.

What Are the Group Leader's Responsibilities?

The group leader plays an important role. Members with no group experiences look to the-leader as a role model — one who sets an example of expected behavior within the group. Members' opinions about a leader are largely based upon her actions. For that reason, a few tips are in order.

1. Be sensitive to others' feelings. The group aims to promote the discovery, expression, and sharing of feelings. The leader encourages others to share their feelings for a reasonable-length of time and doesn't interrupt or take control.

2. Avoid a tendency to dominate the group — to think *your* way is the *only* way. Remember, this is a support *group* — not a support *person*. To encourage each member's participation, emphasize the importance of each one's contribution.

3. Summarize topics that are emphasized, and comment on how

the group discussion is going. Examples: "Many of you mentioned your frustrations about physicians who dismiss your symptoms as unimportant. Has anyone else had a different experience? .

"I noticed we spent the major portion of the meeting discussing how we manage chest pains and palpitations. Has this been helpful, or would you like to discuss another topic?"

4. Keep members of the group actively involved. Ask a question of anyone who hasn't spoken. Examples: "Peggy, we have not heard from you. How has your week been? Mark, I'm interested in your reaction to what Sarah just described. What has been your experience?"

On the other hand, what do you say to persons who monopolize the conversation and annoy the group? Take a direct and firm approach. Examples: "Sue, what you say is important. Now, let us hear from other group members and get *their* opinions.

"Bob, your experience is interesting and helpful. Thank you. I sense other members wait to add to the discussion, and we encourage each one of you to contribute." (If no one volunteers, ask a question and call upon someone.)

Be prepared for the disruptive member. Example: "What's the use of talking about it? I hear the same complaint over and over."

Remind this person it's what *he* brings to the group and expresses that generates power. Each member is responsible for his own contributions.

Show respect for people's personal commitments. Always begin and end meetings on time. Members may be justifiably angry if they've moved mountains to be punctual and meetings both begin and end late. Furthermore, people may feel compelled to stay later than planned, or feel uncomfortable leaving before everyone else.

Ten or fifteen minutes before closing, let members know the meeting is soon ending. Example: "Since it's almost 8:00 P.M., does anyone have a question, or does anyone wish to quickly discuss something?" This is a good time to recap issues, take care of unfinished business, and announce time and place of the next meeting.

What Are Members Responsibilities?

- Arrive on time.

- Understand the purpose and objectives of the group.

- Listen to and show respect for other people's experiences.

- Encourage others to speak. Don't dominate the group.

- Respect all confidential information.

- Own your feelings. Use the pronoun I — *not we* — when you talk about yourself.

- Share the responsibility for making the group work.

How Do I Keep the Group Going Well for an Extended Period of Time?

First, establish purpose, goals, and objectives.

✓ How often, how long, and when should a support group meet? A support group may meet weekly, semimonthly, or monthly from one to two hours depending upon the group's immediate needs. Keep in mind that enthusiasm is often short lived, and weekly meetings sometimes quickly lead to burn out.

The support group of The MVP Program of Cincinnati meets the third Wednesday of the month. The first meting in 1988 was an hour long, and — at members' requests — changed to one-and-a-half hours. It works well for us.

To decide *when* to schedule meetings, select a day and a time that is convenient for the majority of members. Propose a week night or a nontraditional time such as a Saturday brunch. A brunch may enable mothers with baby-sitter problems and any-one who doesn't drive at night to attend. Be flexible.

Identify goals of the group. Are goals short-term or long-term?

✓ What are *your* needs and concerns? Within this group which concerns do we commonly share?

Why did *you* come to this meeting? (On a flip chart, write members' responses for reference. As a leader, be cautious. Do not assume that *you* know all the needs. Remember, all answers are neither right nor wrong and are worthy of discussion.)

Follow through, therefore, and discuss members' concerns to determine additional objectives. You may always add more as you go along. Write all objectives as *positive statements*. Examples: Through this group we'll learn how to deal with our fears. Together we aim to better educate the public about MVPS. We shall share as much information as possible from lectures, from journals, and from this book.

Periodically review objectives. Note any changes in focus within the original group and promptly act. What first began as a sharing of information by members may change. Now, members may wish to become better informed though lectures by knowledgeable people in the medical field. In any event, be alert to the group's wishes. Act accordingly, and don't allow the group to stagnate.

Determine acceptable ground rules

✓ Be sure that all rules are clear and agreeable to each member. For example: Everyone has a right to speak while others politely listen without interrupting. Every speaker rightfully expects confidentiality within the group. We succeed only if *we trust each other*. This is extremely important. Let there be no misconceptions regarding the group's purpose.

Encourage input from _all_ members — both new and old.

✓ Remember to always welcome new members. Ask them to introduce themselves and briefly tell when they were first diagnosed, what symptoms they have, and how they help themselves. Expect some to say, "Gosh, does that sound familiar."

Be careful, however, to avoid the pitfall of the core-group members becoming a clique. The welcoming of new members is a process that continues well beyond welcoming them at the door. Consider a follow-up phone call to new members. How did they like the meeting? Do they plan on attending again? If not, why?

In time, the support group becomes a combination of new and old members; that's good. New members benefit from long-term members' experiences. Likewise, long-term members benefit by learning about recent practices and procedures from new members.

Invite long-term members who are symptom free — and who otherwise may drop out — to remain active and serve as role models. By all means, try to involve them as group facilitators. Ask them to speak at meetings and offer suggestions based upon their own experiences. Members attentively listen to someone who has already "walked in *their* shoes."

Encourage discussion. Ask questions to help members share, think about, and learn from each other's experiences and insights.

EXAMPLES:

Who were most supportive to me in helping me deal with MVPS? What have they said or done that helps me the most?

Who were least supportive? What have they said or done that has not helped?

What should I say in a note or a letter to someone who is facing what I faced?

What is the worst problem that I must face with MVPS?

What problems related to MVPS have I faced and overcome? What problems have I failed to deal with and why?

How did MVPS control my life? In what ways have I learned how to take control?

If I have learned something special about life or human nature as a result of my situation, what is it?

Ensure a Sense of Belonging. Form Committees.

Prepare a list of proposed committees on a flip chart. Leave enough free space underneath each one to write names. Briefly discuss the duties of each committee, length of time each committee serves, and rotation of responsibilities.

Next, either alphabetically assign members to each committee, or ask for volunteers. (To *assign* members may be more effective. We all know the "let-George-do-it type." Do remember, however, to ensure the group's success, see that each member feels needed and respected. Therefore, encourage each one to assume some responsibility as a committee member.) As a group leader, carefully choose a chairperson of each committee — someone who appears to be outgoing and responsible.

Finance Committee. You'll need money for postage, paper, refreshments, and other incidentals. Dues may be necessary, but don't assume everyone can afford to pay. It's possible, therefore, that you may solicit donations from a local organization or business. Examples: A supermarket or a bakery may donate snacks. A printing place may donate scrap paper for fliers.

Recruitment and Retention Committee. To encourage attendance, telephone each member at least one week before every meeting. Ask whether or not each member plans to attend. Then, notify refreshment committee how many to prepare for. On the other hand, be prepared to contact members when meetings are canceled. A telephone tree is helpful. Sally calls two members; these two call two others, and so it goes.

Develop a phone network, or an *MVP Hotline*. Encourage the exchange of telephone numbers to provide members with help by phone when it's needed between meetings. Be certain to include the time of day each member can be called.

To recruit new members, continue to spread the word. Post fliers and advertise in local papers. Be careful, however, to prevent burnout — or undue stress on any one member. List *two* contact persons on all publicity material. This is particularly true for groups who receive many calls.

Refreshment Committee. Solicit food and beverages from members on a rotating basis. Remind members to bring appropriate foods — no caffeinated beverages or chocolate-glazed doughnuts.

Expect the group to experience regular ups and downs in both attendance and enthusiasm. It's natural and to be expected. You'll find this to be true particularly during summer months. Consider meeting every other month, and return to monthly meetings in the fall.

As group leader you may want to join or form a coalition or association of leaders from the same or similar types of self-help groups, for mutual support and for sharing successful program ideas.

How Do I Terminate a Support Group

Expect the life spans of support groups to vary. Some groups at their inception specify a definite number of weeks or months in which to achieve their objectives. For them, termination is expected and accepted.

On the other hand, some groups form stronger bonds and continue to meet month after month, year after year. For these members, the thought of disbanding sometimes poses problems.

Either way, ending need not be a gloomy affair. Instead, let it signal a new *beginning*. Now that you better understand MVPS, you deal with it, and you take control.

Keep in mind that you want members to leave with a sense of satisfaction and closure. At the last meeting, therefore, review and discuss original objectives. Next, evaluate accomplishments versus shortcomings.

For example, ask yourselves the following questions. What progress have you made as an individual or as a group? What have you learned from each other? How did you feel when you first attended a meeting? How do you feel now? What concerns do you still have? Can you cope with MVPS more satisfactorily? If so, in what way? To answer these questions puts your goals in-perspective. Thus, you focus on *achievements*.

During the period óf termination, remember several house-keeping items. Pay outstanding bills. Return borrowed supplies or equipment. Notify and thank sponsors, referral agencies, who-ever furnished a meeting room, as well as anyone else who helped. Explain that your group accomplished its objectives and terminates on *(date)* . In this way, you leave the door open for future groups who may wish to be accommodated.

Finally, when your group disbands, write the names, addresses, and phone numbers of newly made friends. Keep in touch. For, as a song popular during the 1960's goes:

"I get by with a little help from my friends."

MVP Support Groups

If you start or terminate a support group, let The MVPPC know. Please call (513) 745-9911.

Alabama

Carol Arnold
P.O. Box 582
Anniston, AL 36202

Jan Black
122 Snowden Circle
Birmingham, AL 35235
(205) 655-2377

Pepper Hoover
Cullman Regional Medical Center
1912 Alabama Highway 157
Cullman, AL 35056
(205) 737-2593

Gina Willis
2107 Serene Path
Leeds, AL 35094
(205) 299-7813

Alaska

Loretta Fitzgerald
15721 Southpark Loop
Anchorage, AK 99516
(907) 345-8750

American On-Line Computer Network:

Christine Critelli Earley, from Lyndhurst, New Jersey has started an MVP support group on line.
Here is how to access the group:
Keyword "Health"; Click on "Message Center"
Click on "List Categories"
Click on "Self-Help & Support Groups"
Click on "Mitral Valve Prolapse Syndrome"
Meetings are bi-weekly on Mondays at 11:00 P.M. EST.
Contact Christine at chrissi580@aol.com

California

Meredith Boyd
Central California Chapter
163 Ramona Drive
San Luis Obispo, CA
(805) 544-0545

Pat Bringel
38 Heather Lane
Orinda, CA 94563
(510) 254-0183

Jane Emmer
1460 7th Street, Suite 301
Santa Monica, CA 90401

National Society for MVP/Dysautonomia
Los Angeles Chapter, 1st Tuesday at 7:15 P.M. at
Faith Community Church
15906 E. San Bernardino Rd.
Covina, CA 91722
Call Alicia Vaughn (213) 256-3574 or
Catherine Thomas (818) 798-3466

Karen Rayburn
Monrovia, CA
(818) 359-4974

Catherine Thomas
3232 Barhite Street
Pasadena, CA 91107
(818) 798-3466

Susie Warman
15 Via De La Mesa
RSM, CA 92688

Colorado

Laura Lewis
5335 Holmes Place
Bolder, CO 80303
(303) 447-1191

Andrea Shaw
36 Luxury Lane
Colorado Springs, CO 80921
(719) 488-3244

Connecticut

Lou Ann Glazer
98 Ocean Drive
Stamford, CT 06902
(203) 357-7577

Florida

Robin Cantwell
2617 Country Club Road
Eustis, FL 32726
(904) 357-4409

Kathleen Christiansen
Florida Hospital Center for Women's Medicine
2501 North Orange, Suite 340
Lakeland, FL 32803
(813) 646-6609

Judy Hunter
Orlando Women's Medical Center
Orlando, FL 32803
(407) 896-6611

Mary Ann Kailing
2158 Victory Garden
Tallahassee, FL 32301
(904) 877-0549

Elaine Klein
5555 Collins Avenue, Apt. 10M
Miami Beach, FL 33140

Jeanette Phillip
6705 Southwest 44th St., Apt 58
Miami, FL 33155
(305) 661-7817
CompuServe mail code: 73252,1447

Jean Tomany
206 2nd Street East
Bradenton, FL 34208
(813) 746-5111

Georgia

Amy Poe
1885 Meadowchase Court
Snellville, GA 30278
(770) 979-5348

Kathie Scott
2102 Memorial Drive #45
Waycross, GA 31501

Nancy Tkaczuk
Northside Medical Center
1000 Johnson Ferry Road
Atlanta, GA 30342
(404) 851-8000

Illinois

Coleen Bennett
302½ South Gridley
Bloomington, IL 61701
(309) 829-8438

Carol Hegberg
936 North 12th Street
Dekalb, IL 60115
(815) 756-2520

Linda Kyk
St. Joe area of Chicago
(815) 726-1917

Lorette Levine
Suburban Medical Center
Chicago, IL

MVP Support Group
800 Biesterfield
Elk Grove, IL 60143
Alexian Brothers Medical Center; Meets 3rd Tuesday at 7:00 P.M.
Send long self-addressed, stamped envelope to: MVP Support
Group. P.O. Box 431, Itasca, IL 60143-0431

Ann Tucker
Good Samaritan Hospital
3815 Highland Ave
Downers Grove, IL 60515
(708) 719-4799

Indiana

State of Indiana, MVP Support Group
Heart Center of Fort Wayne
7836 W. Jefferson Blvd.
Fort Wayne, IN 46802
(219) 432-2297

Maryland

Francine T. Marsili
6924 Meadowlake Road
New Market, MD 21774
(301) 865-0425

Massachusetts

Carole Kerber
1500 Worcester Road
Framingham, MA 01701
(508) 879-8124

Michigan

Barb Astalos
21405 Danbury Drive
Woodhaven, MI 48183
(313) 671-8987

Susan Vogt
13550 Moceri Circle
Warren, MI 48093
(810) 978-1568

New Jersey

Donna Dewedoff
305 Jane Road
Cinnominson, NJ 08077
(609) 786-0995

Cynthia Suchowacki, RN
91 West 3rd Street
Bayonne, NJ 07002

New York

Barbar Boeck
365 North 7th Street
Lewiston, NY 14902
(716) 754-7549

Joan Cohn, DSW
Associate Director Mental Health
Womens Health Promotion
Mt. Sinai Medical Center
5 East 98 Street
New York, NY 10029
(212) 241-3249   Fax (212)410-5777

North Carolina

Louise Hyatt
1308 Danbury Court
High Point, NC 27262
(910) 855-4602

Western North Carolina MVPS and Dysautonomia Support
Diane Stepkoski
15 White Squirrel Lane
Hendersonville, NC 28739
(704) 692-6246

Ohio

Tonya Emaheiser
16040 Deshler Road
N. Baltimore, OH 45872
(419) 257-2190

Rosemary Hurley-Jones
4098 Wagner Road
Dayton, OH 45540
(513) 429-5282

Kristine A. Scordo, PhD, RN
MVP Program of Cincinnati
10525 Montgomery Road
Cincinnati, OH 45242
(513) 745-9911 for information

Debbie Stires
3515 Harrison NW
Canton, OH 44709

Oklahoma

Becky Dunn
P.O. Box 1805
Ft. Gibson, OK 74434
(918) 478-3185

Pennsylvania

Mary Matalon
Cardiac Rehab
Lancaster General Hospital
554 North Duke Street
Lancaster, PA 17604
(717) 295-8495

Carolyn Mitreiber
736 Linden Street
Bethlehem, PA 18018
(215) 974-8172

Carol Schneider
1866 Warriors Road
Pittsburg, PA 15205

Prodigy®

MVP support group.
Sign on, Jump (F₆) and type *medical support bb*. Under *Choose Topic*, select *Heart Disease*. Type *MVP*; back date to read previous notes.

South Carolina

Melissa Taube
201 Williamsburg Drive
Greer, SC 29651
(803) 879-0845

Tennessee

Dee Dee Meadows
2521 Jeffrey Drive
Chattanooga, TN 37421
(615) 892-3498

Texas

Shirley Burgett
P.O. Box 241
McQueeney, TX 78123
(210) 560-3464

Sandy Haddock
8406 Sageline
San Antonio, TX 78251
(210) 681-7817

Diana Krug
MVPS&D Association
P.O. Box 1641
Pearland, TX 77588
(713) 997-9657
or Margie Oden (713) 334-3733

Dixie Smith
San Antonio, TX
(210) 490-7524

Virginia

Rose Mary Berger
1330 Vanetta Lane
Vienna, VA 22182
(703) 759-5979

Elly Brosius
P.O. Box 1872
Herndon, VA 20172

Wayne Browning
Route 2, Box 138A
Clintwood, VA 24228
(703) 926-6729

Janet Mercadante
3920 Shady Oak Drive
Virginia, Beach, VA 23455
Work: (804) 640-4336   Home: (804) 460-3239

Sharon Utz, PhD, RN
University of Virginia
Charlottesville, VA 22903-3395
(814) 924-0081
Group meets on the first Wednesday from 7:30 to 9 P.M. at the
School of Nursing, McLeod Hall

Washington

Marie Lagerquist
9136 173rd Avenue S.W.
Rochester, WA 98579

References

Govaerts, K. 1991. "Starting a support group." *Diabetes Forecast.* 54–60.

Nichols, K. & Jenkinson, J. 1991. *Leading a Support Group.* Chapman and Hall. London.

Toseland, R., & Rivas, R. 1984. *An Introduction to Group Work Practice.* MacMillan Publishing Comapny. New York.

Utz, S. W. 1994. "Helpful hints for facilitating suport groups." Personal communication.

White, B. & Madara, E. 1992. *The Self-help Sourcebook: Finding & Forming Mutal Aid Self-help Groups.* 4th edit. St. Clares-Riverside Medical Center. Denville, New Jersey.

7

Medication Treatment for MVPS

The purpose of this chapter is to *briefly* highlight information about medications commonly used with MVPS. The intent is not to recommend one drug over another, or to recommend any medication. In fact, many MVPers do well *without* medications. Others *require* medication for symptom control. Therefore, *always* discuss the need for medication with your physician.

Remember, medications don't *cure* MVPS. Unlike a kidney infection, for which you take an antibiotic to effect a *cure*, medication for MVPS is prescribed *to lessen the intensity, or frequency of debilitating symptoms*. For example: Some MVPers take medication for frequent palpitations that cause syncope — temporary loss of consciousness. Others take medication to prevent migraine headaches. Many MVPers take prescribed beta blockers to relieve chest pains and palpitations. Others don't. In spite of beta blockers, they continue to be symptomatic.

A complete list of medications, side effects, and drug interactions, are beyond the scope of this book. If you're interested in further information about medication, see references at the end of this chapter, or consult your nurse, physician, or pharmacist. For a discussion of medications used for the treatment of anxiety and panic attacks, see Chapter 5.

Beta-Blocking Agents

The group of drugs commonly prescribed for symptomatic MVPS are beta blockers. These drugs may prevent migraine headaches and may alleviate symptoms such as chest pain and palpitations.

As you learned in Chapter 1, catecholamines — epinephrine, norepinephrine — regulate many bodily responses. Effects of catecholamines depend upon their interactions with specific receptors located on cell membranes. Receptors recognize catecholamines, allow these substances to interact with the cell, and cause varying physiological responses.

To simplify an explanation of how catecholamines — epinephrine and norepinephrine — interact to regulate bodily responses, see the following analogy.

Your daughter's new date — norepinephrine — comes to your house — a cell. Norepinephrine rings the doorbell. You let him in, since you are a receptor and as a receptor, you recognize a catecholamine. One look at this scruffy character — norepinephrine — and you faint. He caused a physiological response in you, the receptor.

Two types of receptors within the sympathetic nervous system are alpha and beta. Alpha receptors are located in blood vessels throughout the body. Stimulation of alpha receptors by catecholamines — epinephrine and norepinephrine — causes constriction or narrowing of blood vessels. Beta receptors are divided into the $beta_1$ receptors found in heart muscle, and the beta receptors found in the heart muscle and the bronchial — lung, and vascular smooth muscle.

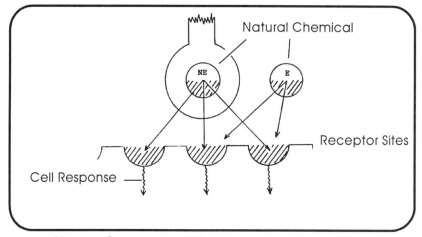

NATURAL CHEMICALS: NE-NOREPINEPHRINE; E-EPINEPHRINE

Stimulation of beta receptors in the heart causes an increase in heart rate, and strengthens the heart muscle's contraction. Stimulation of receptors in vascular smooth muscle causes blood vessels to dilate. Drugs that *block* the action of these receptors are called *beta blockers*.

Beta *blockers* block actions of the sympathetic nervous system — the accelerator. To do this, they block the action of catecholamines — epinephrine and norepinephrine. The pharmacological-properties determine the precise action of the drug. Predictable effects of beta blockers include: lowered blood pressure; lowered resting heart rate, as well as lowered heart-rate response during-exercise; a blunt sympathetic nervous system's response to stress; an increase in left ventricular volume — amount of blood in the heart's pumping chamber; and a decrease in the force of the heart's contraction.

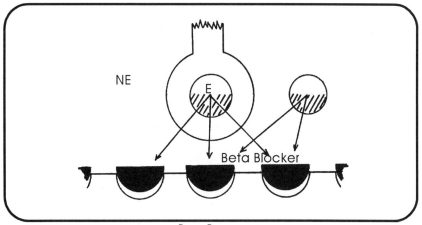

BETA BLOCKER

BETA-BLOCKING AGENTS

- Blockadren (timolol)
- Corgard (nadolol)
- Inderal (propranolol)
- Kerlone (betaxolol)
- Lopressor (metoprolol)
- Sectral(acebutolol)
- Tenormin (atenolol)
- Toprol XL (metoprolol extended release)
- Visken (pindolol)
- Zebeta (bisoprolol fumarate)

How do beta blockers affect your heart rate? Example: Suppose you're physically deconditioned. Your pulse rate at rest is 100 beats per minute. After you climb a flight of stairs, your heart rate increases to 150 beats per minute. Your physician pre-scribes a beta blocker. Now your resting heart rate slows to 60 beats per minute. Again, climb the same flight of stairs at the same pace. With a beta blocker your heart rate increases to *only* 90 rather than 150 beats per minute. Thus, beta blockers atten-uate the heart rate's response to exercise.

Possible side effects of beta blockers include: fatigue, night-mares, mental depression, stomach upset, sexual dysfunction, cold extremities, and wheezing or worsening of asthma. If you experience any of these symptoms, notify your physician.

The peak action of the long-acting beta blockers — Corgard, Kerlone, Tenormin, Toprol XL, Zebeta — occurs two to four hours after taken. This may cause fatigue and sleepiness. To combat these feelings, take a once-a-day beta blocker in the *evening*.

Beta blockers may interact with other medications. Aluminum salts found in some antacids, and cholesterol-lowering medica-tions such as Colestid — colestipol and Questran — cholestyramine, may decrease the absorption of beta blockers. Therefore, be *sure* to take these medications at *least two hours* after you take a beta blocker. Similarly, food may alter the avail-ability of the drug absorbed in the stomach. Therefore, establish a pattern, and regularly take the medication either with or with-out food. This helps to minimize any variation in absorption.

Digitalis

Digitalis — digoxin, digitoxin, Lanoxin, Lanoxicaps — is usually given to MVPers with arrhythmias such as PSVT — paroxysmal supraventricular tachycardia, and atrial fibrillation.-Digitalis slows the heart rate; slows electrical conduction to prevent excessive impulses from being conducted to the ventricles; and strengthens the force of the heart's contraction.

Digitalis preparations have a variety of drug interactions. For example: antacids, bran, antibiotics — neomycin, sulfasalazine — and some cholesterol-lowering agents — Questran, Colestid — decrease the absorption of digitalis. Since these interactions decrease the amount available for the body's use, don't take any of the above-mentioned medications *together*. Instead, take each medication *two hours apart*. On the other hand, some antibiotics — erythromycin and tetracycline — *can increase* the amount of digitalis in the body. Also, many drugs interfere with the excre-tion of digitalis. *Always notify your physician if any additional medications are ever prescribed for you.*

An initial sign that there's too much digitalis in your system is a loss of appetite sometimes followed by nausea and vomiting. Other side effects may include headache, fatigue, drowsiness, and generalized muscle weakness. If any of these symptoms occur, notify your physician.

Calcium Channel Blockers

To varying degrees, calcium channel blockers affect the heart rate, electrical conduction, and the tone of the arterial and venous blood vessels. From this group of drugs, Diltiazem and Verapamil are used primarily for the management of arrhythmias and migraine headaches. Verapamil or Diltiazem, either by themselves or in combination with digitalis or beta blockers, can be helpful in the management of atrial fibrillation, or paroxysmal supraventricular tachycardia-(PSVT).

These drugs are usually well tolerated, but side effects are possible. They may include: constipation, dizziness, lightheadedness, and swelling of ankles or legs.

CALCIUM CHANNEL-BLOCKING AGENTS

- Cardizem, Dilacor (diltiazem)
- Cardene (nicardipine)
- Dynacirc (isradipine)
- Isoptin, Verelan, Calan (verapamil)
- Nimotop (nimodipine)
- Norvasc (amlodipine)
- Plendil (felodipine)
- Procardia, Adalat (nifedipine)
- Vascor (bepridil)

Antiarrhythmic Drugs

This group of drugs is used to treat MVPers with ventricular arrhythmias — abnormalities of the heart's rhythm that originate from the heart's lower chambers. Before these drugs are used, two critical questions must be answered. One, is the arrhythmia serious enough to require therapy, and two, which specific drug should be used?

The answer to the first question includes MVPers who have arrhythmias that cause syncope — temporary loss of consciousness. This small group is usually treated with medication. A larger group of people experience palpitations or skipped beats. Although usually benign, the arrhythmia disrupts each one's general well-being and causes undue anxiety. For these MVPers, antiarrhythmics may be indicated. Although beta blockers are commonly used, antiarrhythmics such as Pronestyl — procainamide, Quinidex — quinidine, Norpace — disopyramide and Mexitil — mexiletine may be prescribed.

Summary

Because many MVPers are young, and medications have side effects, long-term drug therapy is usually avoided. Most physicians recommend that MVPers become more knowledgeable and learn to rely more on non-drug interventions to decrease their symptoms.

Questions Commonly Asked about Medications

1. Do I have to take medication for MVPS for the remainder of my life?

This depends on why the medication was originally prescribed. If, for example, you presently take medication because you have experienced episodes of passing out due to arrhythmia, most likely you must continue the medication. If, however, you take medication for other symptoms — chest pain or headache — you may be able to discontinue the medication. Many MVPers take medication, particularly a beta blocker, only prior to and during stressful situations that increase their symptoms. Discuss this with your physician.

Many people experience symptoms even with medications. Others cannot tolerate the side-effects. There are those MVPers who prefer not to take any medication. As one of our MVP Program participants said, "Before I joined the program, I experienced fatigue, extra heart beats, and chest pains. Although I took a beta blocker, my symptoms continued. Now that I want to get-pregnant, I avoid taking any form of medication. Instead, with exercise, proper diet, and relaxation techniques, I weaned myself off the beta blocker. Furthermore, I even feel better now than I did before."

A note of caution: Do not stop taking any medication till you discuss it with your physician. Also be sure you know *why* each medication is prescribed. For example, will it control chest pains, or is it prescribed for other reasons.

2. What should I ask my physician about my medications?

For various reasons, many MVPers hesitate to question their physician about prescribed medications. "He's too busy. He will think my question is stupid. I'm not sure what to ask." To correctly take a prescribed medication — know *what* you'll take and *why*, *when* to take it, and *whether side effects are possible.* Take notes, and don't leave the physician's office till you fully understand. If you think of additional questions later on, write them down and either *call* the physician's office, or *wait* until your next visit.

3. Is it true you can't benefit from exercise if you take a beta blocker?

MVPers who take beta blockers often believe they can't obtain a *training effect* — or benefit from cardiovascular exercise — because beta blockers lower resting rate and exercise heart rate — two indicators of a training effect. This, however, is not entirely true.

You'll recall from Chapter 4 that cardiovascular exercise offers many benefits. The extent of the training effect, however, depends upon many factors. These include: your initial level of fitness; type and dosage of beta blocker; frequency, duration, and intensity of exercise. The results of a graded-exercise stress test — proof of effectiveness of cardiovascular training — depend upon whether the initial test and follow-up test were both performed while you took a beta blocker.

If you take a beta blocker, don't try to achieve a target heart rate. To increase your heart rate to such a level requires high-intensity exercise. This is unnecessary and not recommended. You'll easily tire, exercise less, and enjoy very little benefit from exercise. Instead, use the Borg scale of perceived exertion, and exercise only to a perception of *somewhat hard.* That's sufficient. Although it may take longer to achieve a training effect, *it will happen.*

PRACTICAL GUIDELINES FOR DRUG TREATMENT

- Take your medications at the same times each day.
- If you miss a dose, do not double the next scheduled dose.
- Carry a list of your medications or a medication card in your wallet or purse.
- List both the trade and generic names of the drugs.
- Before having surgery — including dental surgery, or emergency treatment, notify the- physician of your medications.
- If you are either pregnant, or plan to become pregnant, or are breast feeding, let your physician know before you take medications. Medications may have an adverse effect on the fetus. They may also pass into the breast milk and cause unwanted effects in the infant.
- When you travel, carry enough medication with you to last a few days in case your luggage is misplaced; or in the event your trip is unexpectedly lengthened.
- Keep drugs in their original containers to maintain the drugs' potency.
- Keep original labels on the drug's container.
- Store medications in a cool, dry place, out of direct sunlight. A medicine cabinet in a warm, humid bathroom, a glove compartment or a car's trunk — particularly during warmer weather — are *poor* storage places.
- *Never* share prescriptive medications with friends. Others may be allergic to the drug, or they *may not* have the same problem, and react differently.
- *Never* take medications in darkness because bottles and pills look alike. Serious errors are possible.
- *Never* swallow medications while lying down.
- Don't put more than one medication in a bottle.
- Always ask a pharmacist or other health professional how to take medications. To crush or chew a pill may alter its reaction in the body.
- Always read labels for proper administration of the drug, and for drug interactions.

PRACTICAL GUIDELINES FOR DRUG TREATMENT

- Regularly, clean out your medication cabinet. Over time, moisture, heat and light degrade medications and render them less active. In some cases, decomposed medication becomes a dangerous drug. Therefore, dispose of outdated drugs, old prescriptive medications with no expiration dates; unidentifiable medicine; cracked, chipped or discolored tablets; and capsules that have softened, cracked, or stuck together. Flush unsafe medications down the toilet. Never throw them in a waste-paper basket or a garbage pail.

REFERENCES

About Your Medications. 1986. The United States Pharmacopeial Convention, Inc. Rockville, MD.

Boudoulas, H. & Wooley, C. 1988. "Mitral valve prolapse syndrome: Therapeutic considerations." In: *Mitral Valve Prolapse and the Mitral Valve Prolapse Syndrome* (H. Boudoulas & C. Wooley, Eds.). 555–563.

Clayman, C. (Ed.) 1988. *The American Medical Association Guide to Prescription and over-the-Counter Drugs*. Random House. New York.

Frishman, W. 1984. *Clinical Pharmacology of the B-adrenoceptor Blocking Drugs*. 2nd edit. Appleton-Century-Crofts. Norwalk, CT.

Griffin, J., D'Arcy, P., & Speirs, C. 1988. *A Manual of Adverse Drug Interactions*. Wright. London.

Hansten, P. & Horn, J. (1989). *Drug Interactions*. 6th edit. Lea & Febiger. Philadelphia.

Harvard Medical School Health Letter. March, 1989, 14, 5.

Katzung, B. (Ed.). 1989. *Basic and Clinical Pharmacology*. 4th edit. Appleton & Lange. Norwalk, CT.

McEvoy, G. (Ed.) 1990. American Hospital Formulary Service Drug Information 90. American Society of Hospital Pharmacists, Inc. Bethesda, MD.

Opie, L. (Ed.) 1995. *Drugs for the Heart*. 4th edit. Grune & Stratton, Inc. New York.

Reiser, J. & Horowitz, L. (Eds.) 1985. *Mechanisms and Treatment of Cardiac Arrhythmias: Relevance of Basic Studies to Clinical Management*. Urban & Schwarzenberg. Baltimore-Munich.

Saltissik, S., et al. 1983. "The effects of oral digoxin therapy in primary mitral leaflet prolapse." *The European Society of Cardiology*. **4**: 828–837.

Frequently Asked Questions about MVPS

Since the publication of the first edition of *Taking Control*, we received countless letters from people all over the world. A compilation of common questions from people who wrote *Network's* column, the Readers' Corner, follows.

How Important Is it to Take Antibiotics, and Why Take Them?

Although MVPS is a relatively benign condition, one possible complication is infective endocarditis (IE). Infective endocarditis is a bacterial infection of the heart valve(s) or lining of the heart. It occurs when bacteremia — bacteria in the bloodstream — lodge on an abnormal heart valve or other damaged tissue. In MVP, mechanical stress and turbulent blood flow may injure a valve's surface and create an opportunity for bacteria in the blood stream to deposit on the valve. The bacteria cause wart-like growths that can damage, and even destroy the heart valve.

Certain heart conditions place a person at a greater risk for developing endocarditis when a bacteremia occurs. Some of these conditions include:

- prosthetic — artificial heart valves
- certain congenital — birth — cardiac malformations
- valvular heart disease — such as valves damaged by rheumatic fever and other acquired valve dysfunction
- mitral valve prolapse with regurgitation — back flow of blood through the opening of the mitral valve leaflets
- hypertrophic cardiomyopathy — heart muscle disease
- people who have previously had bacterial endocarditis, even in the absence of heart disease

Bacteria commonly enter the bloodstream during certain surgical procedures that involve-contaminated tissue, and during dental procedures that may cause gingival — gum — bleeding. This causes a transient — a brief — bacteremia that rarely lasts for more than 15 minutes. Only a limited number of types of bacteria commonly cause endocarditis. It is impossible to predict, however, which person will develop an infection — or which particular procedure will be responsible. Unless there are antibiotics in the blood to combat the bacteria, this bacteremia can cause endocarditis.

Since the 1950's, The American Heart Association — AHA — has published guidelines for the prevention of bacterial endocarditis. The latest guidelines were published in *JAMA, December 12, 1990.* In general, antibiotic prophylaxis is recommended for all dental procedures likely to cause gingival bleeding, even for routine professional cleaning. Antibiotics are also recommended for surgery, instrumentation, or diagnostic procedures that involve the genitourinary or gastrointestinal tracts, such as: gallbladder surgery, bronchoscopy, and incision and drainage of infected tissue.

PROCEDURES FOR WHICH ENDOCARDITIS PROPHYLAXIS IS INDICATED INCLUDE (Dajani et al., 1990):

- Dental procedures known to induce gingival — gum — bleeding including professional cleaning (not simple adjustment of orthodontic appliances or natural loss of a tooth)
- Tonsillectomy and/or adenoidectomy
- Surgical procedures or biopsy involving respiratory mucosa
- Bronchoscopy with a rigid bronchoscope
- Sclerotherapy of esophageal varices
- Esophageal dilatation
- Gallbladder surgery
- Cystoscopy
- Urethral dilatation
- Urethral catheterization if urinary tract infection present
- Prostatic surgery
- Incision and drainage of infected tissue
- Vaginal hysterectomy
- Vaginal delivery in the presence of infection

The recommended standard drug for all *dental, oral, and upper respiratory tract procedures* is amoxicillin. To be effective, 3.0 grams of amoxicillin should be taken by mouth one hour before the procedure; then 1.5 grams are taken six hours after the initial dose. Therefore, if you took the first dose at 8:00 AM, the second dose would be at 2:00 PM. For people who are allergic to penicillins — such as amoxicillin, ampicillin, or penicillin — erythromycin is used. The dose is 800 mgm of erythromycin ethylsuccinate, or 1.0 gram of erythromycin stearate by mouth two hours before the procedure: then half the dose six hours after the initial dose. (For individuals who cannot tolerate either penicillins or erythromycin, clindamycin hydrochloride 300 mgm by mouth 1 hour before the procedure and 150 mgm 6 hours after can be used.) Antibiotic prophylaxis is also recommended for children with MVP. The dose of antibiotic is based on the weight of the child. Usually, children over 30 kg (66 pounds) receive the full, adult dose of amoxicillin.

How Do You Know if You Need Antibiotics?

First, and foremost — always verify this with your physician.

Usually this is discussed when you are first diagnosed. The AHA recommends antibiotics for people with MVP and valvular regurgitation or insufficiency — a back flow of blood. This back flow of blood causes a murmur — an extra heart sound. Regurgitation is visible on a color flow — 2D — echocardiographic examination. Therefore, people with MVP who have a murmur should take antibiotics prophylactically. Studies implicate other features associated with MVP. Because these features may increase the risk for developing bacterial endocarditis, many physicians recommend antibiotics if on the echocardiogram, they note thickened or redundant valve leaflets. Others recommend antibiotics if you have a click, or extra heart sound. Recommendations for antibiotic prophylaxis for MVP continue to be controversial; the recommendations are still evolving.

Again, always consult your physician to verify the need for antibiotics.

HELPFUL TIPS WHEN TAKING ANTIBIOTICS

- Obtain the handy wallet-size card from your local chapter of the American Heart Association or physician's office. The card lists the antibiotics and dosage commonly prescribed. Ask your physician to circle the one he recommends, and also list your diagnosis in the space provided. Complete the top of the card with your name, address, and telephone number. Carry this card with you.

- Before any procedure, ask about the need for taking antibiotics. Not every procedure requires them.

- Take the antibiotic on an empty stomach to increase the absorption in the small intestine.

- If you experience stomach upset, nausea, or vomiting when taking amoxicillin, take it with a little food or milk to buffer it. Be sure to check with the dentist to see if you are allowed a small amount of food.

- If your stomach is upset from Erythromycin, get the kinder enteric coated form.

- Antacids decrease drug absorption. Do not take them with antibiotics.

- Alert your physician, pharmacist, nurse to all medications you take — especially if you plan to be on antibiotics any length of time. Many drugs interact with antibiotics.

- To avoid diarrhea, take Lactobacillus tablets — available in many health food stores — or eat four to eight ounces of yogurt daily. Be certain the yogurt contains *live yogurt cultures*. Some refrigerated brands contain live cultures. Frozen yogurt does not.

- Maintain good oral hygiene, and see your dentist regularly. When bleeding occurs with tooth brushing, bacteria that enter the blood stream are usually not sufficient to cause endocarditis. It is, however, important to not let the bacteria build up in your mouth. Brush and floss on a regular basis.

- Report symptoms such as: malaise, fatigue, loss of appetite, fever, or weight loss. These are common symptoms of endocarditis, and they usually start within two weeks of the precipitating bacteremia.

Can People with MVP Safely Use Water Picks to Clean Their Teeth? Would Some Gum Bleeding Be Safe during the Use of this Device?

Water picks are small hoses that produce streams of water to irrigate teeth and supporting structures. Although a water pick *does not* take the place of brushing and flossing, it cleans well around fixed bridges and helps maintain good oral hygiene.

To answer the question: Yes, people with MVP may brush, floss, and use a water pick *if they* have good oral health.

On the other hand, people with MVP who have periodontal disease — indicated by gum bleeding — must exercise caution. They can inadvertently introduce bacteria into the blood stream by brushing, flossing and using a water pick. It is extremely important, therefore, that MVPers work closely with their dentist.

What Effect Does MVPS Have on Pregnancy?

According to available data and clinical experience, women with MVPS need not anticipate complications during pregnancy. In fact, the frequency of complications is no greater in women with MVP than those without MVP.

Women frequently report an increase in their symptoms during the early part of pregnancy. At approximately two months gestation, however, circulatory blood volume rapidly increases. This expansion of intravascular volume causes symptoms related to a low-circulating blood volume — a forceful heart beat and/or dizziness upon standing — to become less evident. Also, the click and murmur — physical findings associated with MVP — sometimes disappear.

Physicians' recommendations for antibiotic prophylaxis — preventive treatment — sometimes vary. Although available data suggests it, antibiotic prophylaxis may not be necessary for an uncomplicated vaginal delivery, many obstetricians prefer to give it to all women who had a murmur prior to pregnancy.

Because of highly mobile joints associated with MVP, it has been suggested that delivery might be easier. However, no evidence supports this hypothesis.

How Great Is My Risk of Sudden Death?

Clinical studies identify two distinct groups of people with mitral valve prolapse. First, is the younger group — predominantly female individuals in their 30s and 40s — and with symptoms unrelated to valvular dysfunction — the mitral valve prolapse syndrome. Second, is the older group — predominantly male individuals over 50 — with symptoms of valvular dysfunction who frequently require mitral-valve surgery — anatomic MVP. The incidence of sudden death is believed to differ between these two groups.

Mitral Valve Prolapse Syndrome

Thus far, research suggests that sudden death in people with mitral valve prolapse who do not have significant mitral regurgitation — back flow of blood into the left atrium or top chamber — is uncommon. Fewer than a hundred cases have been reported in the literature. Since 4–5% of the population — or close to seven million people — have mitral valve prolapse, the incidence of sudden death is very low.

For comparison, the annual risk of sudden death among the *entire* adult US population is estimated at 300,000 per year, mostly due to coronary artery disease. This translates into an overall incidence of sudden death of 10 to 20/10,000 population, or 0.1–0.2% per year. Compare this to the risk of sudden death for MVPS at 2/10,000 population per year, or .02%. The low risk for sudden death among people with MVPS without significant mitral regurgitation is compatible with the belief that uncomplicated MVPS is inherently a benign — favorable — finding.

Anatomic Mitral Valve Prolapse

The development of significant mitral regurgitation, a complication of *anatomic* MVP, occurs in 2 to 4% of people with mitral valve prolapse. This complication occurs more commonly in men above 50 years. The risk of sudden death in this group, although controversial, is *estimated* at 94 to 188 per 10,000, or 1–2% a year, quite different from those without significant mitral regurgitation. This older group has a higher prevalence of complex ventricular arrhythmias — or disturbances in-the heart's rhythm — along with depressed pumping action of the heart muscle. These complex arrhythmias and depressed-heart function, together with significant mitral regurgitation are believed to place this group of people with MVP at a higher risk for sudden death.

Thus, current studies suggest that, although sudden death does occur, it is uncommon among those with MVPS. Although certain predictors of sudden death are not clearly identified, people who *may* be at a higher risk include: those with a history of recurrent syncope — passing out, a history of sustained supraventricular arrhythmias, complex ventricular arrhythmias — repetitive short runs of extra beats, or a family history of cardiac sudden death. Thus far, no single finding -or combination of findings proves to be a consistent predictor of sudden death.

Will the Valve Have to Be Replaced?

This is a common question. Natural history studies indicate people with MVPS with symptoms unrelated to the valve, have a relatively benign prognosis — a normal life span. They rarely require valve replacement.

Will the extra heart sound or sounds *always* be heard on physical examination?

It is well known that MVP is a very dynamic syndrome. Cardiac auscultation — heart sounds — sometimes vary from one examination to another. Due to changes in blood volume within the heart, either or both the click and murmur, diagnostic of MVP, sometimes may not be heard. Likewise, if you are well hydrated, and on beta blockers or tranquilizers, neither a click nor a murmur may be audible.

Will the Echocardiogram *always* Show the MVP?

An echocardiogram — ultrasound — is used to confirm the diagnosis of MVP. The mitral valve, however, may not be optimally visualized. Sometimes, it is difficult to obtain a clear picture of the valve. At other times, MVP may be present, but not seen on the echocardiogram. This is known as a false-negative result.

Usually, if MVP is seen on the echocardiogram, it will be seen on future tests. Negative findings at a later date may be due to either or both inadequate visualization of the mitral valve, or the use of different diagnostic criteria by the physician reader. Although manifestations of MVP vary from day to day, the use of strict echocardiographic criteria can avoid misdiagnosis, and the uncertainty of knowing whether or not MVP is present.

Do the More Symptoms I Have Mean the Worse the Valve Is?

No. In MVPS, there is no correlation between the amount of symptoms an individual has and the degree to which the valve buckles back.

Is It Safe to Take Birth Control Pills if I Have MVPS?

Birth control pills — BCP — sometimes alter the blood-clotting system and increase the risk of cerebrovascular accidents, such as a stroke. This risk may be increased by concomitant cigarette use, high blood pressure, and the use of birth control pills with high estrogen content.

Although the issue of MVP and BCP is not clearly defined, anyone who has suffered any of the following embolic events would be wise to avoid BCP: cerebral embolism — blood clot to the brain, pulmonary embolism — blood clot to the lungs, or transient ischemic attack — TIA.

What may place an individual with MVP at a higher-than-normal risk for cerebral embolism? A combination of cigarette smoking, severe migraine headaches, thickened mitral valve-leaflets — seen on the echocardiogram — and birth control pills. It is recommended that you discuss this with your physician.

Is it Safe to Donate Blood if I Have MVPS?

For most individuals with MVPS, donating blood is not contraindicated — dangerous or undesirable. On the other hand, those who have severe orthostatic hypotension — lowering of the blood pressure upon standing, or those sensitive to volume depletion, should not give blood.

Before giving blood, however, check with your physician first. If you do donate blood, drink plenty of fluids prior to and after the procedure.

What about Getting Life Insurance? Should I Check Heart Disease?

Unfortunately, not everyone is well versed on MVPS. John Q. Public sees the word — valve — and often associates it with a heart disease that carries a different prognosis. Then, some people find it difficult to obtain insurance. Others sometimes even pay higher rates as high-risk individuals.

You are frequently asked, "Do you have heart disease?" Yes, MVP, a valvular disease, falls under the general heading of heart disease. Likewise, *heart disease* and coronary artery disease, although they differ in meaning, come under the same general heading.

Do you have a heart murmur? Do not assume because of MVP you have a murmur. Many MVPers have a click without a murmur — therefore — ask your physician. Computerized cross referencing between insurance companies and physicians' offices has become sophisticated. Honesty is the best policy.

Next, as you shop around for an insurance policy, carefully read any policy that appeals to you. Contact your insurance agent or the insurance company for answers to questions. In spite of frustrations, continue your search. As an informed consumer who diligently shopped, you'll eventually find the policy that fits your budget and your needs. Also, if necessary, ask your physician to discuss in a short letter MVP and its prognosis. It may help.

Should I Have My Children Checked for MVP?

Often, MVP in children is diagnosed as the result of a routine physical examination. The physician hears a click or murmur. However, silent MVP — normal heart sounds — does occur. An echocardiogram confirms the diagnosis. Follow-up includes yearly physical examinations, echocardiograms, and antibiotic prophylaxis.

To a lesser extent, children and adolescents have symptoms similar to adults. Chest pain, palpitations, and shortness of breath are common. The cause of the symptoms remains unknown.

Remember, children are impressionable. Therefore, assure them their condition is not uncommon, and that it is treatable. Also, children learn by example. Have you seen children playing, pretending to be parents? The experience is enlightening. If the parent stays in bed all day and conveys a feeling of fear, expect children to do so. Strive to be a good role model with healthy attitudes and behavior patterns.

How Can I Be Sure that the Chest Pain Is Not from Coronary Artery Disease?

The answer to this relates to your original diagnosis. To first determine if heart disease is present, your physician considers your cardiovascular risk factors, symptoms, and diagnostic-test results. Periodically follow-up, with testing such as an exercise stress test, reassures you the chest pain is not caused by coronary artery disease.

I Seem to Be More Flexible than Other People. Is this Part of MVPS?

As a child, could you assume a yoga position much easier than your friends? Could you bend your fingers way back and also perform other contortions? Increased joint flexibility, commonly associated with MVP, theoretically relates to a generalized alteration of connective tissue. Connective tissue is found in tendons, ligaments, and muscles. One of its major components is collagen. Collagen — a protein — is a tough, fibrous material that provides strength to various structures within the body. There are a number of different types of collagen. Changes in the composition of these collagen types, found in connective tissue, enhance joint flexibility.

Why Are MVPS Symptoms More Frequent and Intense When I Am Sick with a Cold, Flu, or an Infection?

Various stressors, whether with a physiological basis — such as infection — or with a psychological basis — such as emotional stress — can worsen MVPS symptoms. For example, during menses, many women report their symptoms either intensify or surface more frequently. Stressors, such as arthritic pain or infections, affect a number of bodily systems, one of which is the autonomic nervous system. Over sensitivity of this system is believed to cause a number of the symptoms associated with MVPS.

When you are ill, it is important to continue non-drug symptom control. In other words, maintain an adequate fluid intake. Avoid caffeinated products and medications that contain adrenalinelike substances. Get adequate rest. Do not overexert yourself. Overexertion — particularly when you are ill — prolongs recovery. Once you feel better, begin exercising to a perceived exertion of fairly light. Shortly afterward, gradually increase the intensity of your workload to a perceived exertion of somewhat hard. The better conditioned you are, the easier it becomes to bounce back.

What Medications May I Safely Use when I Have a Cold, or when My Allergies Worsen?

Not all MVPers react the same. Many experience increased symptoms when they use antihistamines or decongestants.

Therefore, never randomly select an over-the-counter medication. But, don't despair. There are prescription medications that offer relief of cold or allergy symptoms without increasing MVPS symptoms.

Antihistamines

Antihistamines are medications that interfere with histamine, a culprit responsible for sneezing, a stuffy nose, a runny nose, and itching eyes, all of which are associated with allergies. Antihistamines prevent rather than reverse the actions of histamines. For maximum effectiveness, take medication one to two hours *before* anticipated exposure to the offending allergen. Example: If you're allergic to cut grass, take an antihistamine at least one hour before you walk in a recently mowed area.

The anticholinergic properties of these drugs cause the drying effects of antihistamines. An anticholinergic blocks or interferes with the action of the parasympathetic nervous system — the-decelerator. For some MVPers, these anticholinergic effects also cause tachycardia — fast heart beat and palpitations. Also, because antihistamines may have a sedative effect, they can cause drowsiness.

Not all antihistamines are alike. Different agents have varying sedative and anticholinergic effects. Antihistamines with little or no central or autonomic nervous system effects are now available. These drugs have either minimal or no sedative or anticholinergic effects. They include: Seldane (terfenadine), Hismanal (astemizole), and Claritin (loratadine). MVPers who noted-increased symptoms with over-the-counter antihistamines, seem to do better with these newer medications.

A word of caution with Seldane and Hismanal. Although *rare*, but because of potential serious cardiovascular adverse events, *do not* take Seldane and Hismanal in combination with the following medications: Nizoral (ketoconazole), Sporanox (itraconazole), Zithromax (azithromycin), Biaxin (clarithromycin), Tao (troleandomycin) and erythromycin. On the other hand, this is not true for Claritin (loratadine). This drug may be taken with the above medications.

Decongestants

Decongestants are sympathomimetic agents. They mimic the action of the sympathetic nervous system — the accelerator. Therefore, they can cause palpitations, a rapid heart beat, and nervous feeling. Unlike antihistamines, these drugs are mostly used to relieve symptoms related to colds and allergies. Studies associated with people not known to have MVPS, report that decongestants with pseudoephedrine hydrochloride are reasonable safe at dosages less than 180 mg. According to studies, in higher doses, however, pseudoephedrine raised blood pressure and heart rate in normal subjects. Although no studies have been conducted in people with MVPS, if you must take a decongestant choose one with the lowest dose of pseudoephedrine hydrochloride.

Is There a Relationship between Symptoms and Work Schedules?

Yes, it's not unusual for symptoms to worsen if your job is very stressful. For example, does it require rotating shifts and long hours? Are you unhappy with your position? If so, learn to help yourself in other ways, such as stress management and non-drug symptom control interventions.

Do Other People with MVPS Complain of Increased Symptoms due to Insufficient Sleep?

Yes. It is not unusual for people with MVPS to complain of sleeplessness caused by insomnia, anxiety, or palpitations. Lack of sleep causes even more fatigue, irritability, and a host of other complaints. Any type of stress — including sleeplessness — can potentially increase symptoms associated with MVPS.

To hasten sleep, avoid eating highly acidic foods, such as tomatoes and citrus fruits, late at night. Also, avoid alcohol — particularly wine. While it quickly brings on sleep, it awakens you in the middle of the night. Furthermore, alcohol, along with insufficient water intake can also lead to dehydration, fatigue, headaches, and disturbed sleep.

Known stimulants such as: caffeine, nicotine, and foods high in sugar also cause sleeplessness. Wind down a few hours before you retire. Relax, watch TV, listen to the radio, or read. Learn *how* to effectively deal with everyday stressors. Also, get regular cardiovascular exercise. Those MVPers who exercise on a regular basis enjoy better sleep patterns.

Does a Person's Weight Have anything to Do with Having Symptoms of MVP?

Thus far, no published studies address a relationship between a person's weight and the degree of MVP symptoms. People of all shapes and sizes suffer from symptoms to varying degrees. From clinical observations, however, thinner people with MVPS frequently have lower blood pressures. Their pressure may further decrease whenever they rise, from either a lying or a sitting position. Then, along with a compensatory increase in heart rate, they feel lightheaded, and they note a forceful heartbeat. This reaction may be partly related to a decreased intravascular volume — the volume of blood contained within the circulatory system.

Theoretically, obesity can worsen MVPS symptoms. Frequently, obese individuals are in poor cardiovascular condition. This leads to higher resting heart rates and inappropriate increases in heart rate with minimal activities. Both contribute to fatigue.

I Know I Am Supposed to Exercise, but How Can I When I'm Exhausted?

Listen to an MVP program participant. "I believe the exercise program greatly improved my MVP symptoms. During the first four weeks of exercise, my symptoms remained constant. I experienced heart palpitations, dizziness, and fatigue daily. I became frustrated, unmotivated, and anxious. I wanted immediate results.

"During the fifth and sixth weeks, I experienced heart palpitations only three or four days each week — not daily.

"As the weeks passed, I became less dizzy as I arose from a seated position. Also, after twelve weeks, I feel less tired by night, and no longer take a lengthy, daily rest. Too, I am less moody and-less irritable.

"In every way, this exercise program offers a positive experience. I am in much better physical condition and in greater control of my MVP symptoms. I highly recommend exercise — it is invaluable."

Remember, Rome was not created in a day. Don't expect miracles over night. Give it time, and you WILL start to feel better.

I Recently Moved. How Can I Find a Physician?

MVPers recommend these ideas:

- Ask friends to help. Someone knows someone else who knows a physician to recommend.

- Call a local hospital and ask to speak to a nurse in the coronary care unit or the cardiac step-down unit. Explain that you are new to the area and in need of a cardiologist. Ask if she would please recommend someone These units tend to be very busy. *Please understand if someone cannot assist you at that moment, ask if you may leave your phone number, or else call again.*

- Contact your local cardiac rehabilitation facility.

- Call the local Academy of Medicine.

- Call a local women's club.

- Speak to people at the YWCA or YMCA.

- Check the local paper for a class or symposium on a heart-health related topic where the speaker is a physician.

- Call your local "Ask a Nurse" program or a physician-referral source. These services are usually organized by local hospitals.

- Call your local Welcome Wagon organization.

- Call the local women's center, such as Women Helping Women, or one at an area hospital.

- Call a local MVP support-group member.

When I Have a Skipped Beat, it Feels like My Heart Stopped. Does it?

No, it doesn't stop.

Skipped or extra beats are very common among MVPers *and* the general public. Premature ventricular contractions — PVCs

— frequently cause this sensation. While some people feel each beat, others are unaware of them. PVCs sometimes occur following the use of caffeine, alcohol, or certain medications. Emotional stress and smoking may also cause PVCs.

Premature ventricular contractions are beats that come ahead of the normal electrical sequence. When a premature beat occurs, the heart doesn't fill with its normal amount of blood. Thus, the contraction is less forceful than normal. To compensate for this early beat, the heart pauses. This pause — a compensatory pause — gives the heart a longer time to fill. What you feel, therefore, is the normal compensatory pause.

When Should a Person, as a Last Alternative, Consider Medication for Heart Palpitations?

The answer to this question depends upon the type of rhythm problem that causes palpitations and your symptoms. With MVP, one treats the symptoms, not the valve. Therefore, unlike antibiotics that cure infections, medications do not cure MVP. Many MVPers reported they continue to have symptoms even with medications. Others said they felt worse after starting medication. No studies support the positive effects of medication on MVP symptoms.

Not all MVPers require medication. Occasional extra beats, or flip-flops, although annoying and frightening, seldom require medication. Consuming adequate amounts of salt and water often alleviates the pounding sensation — or forceful heartbeat — noted upon standing. People with rhythm disturbances, however, such as atrial fibrillation, or episodes of passing out due to-arrhythmias — disturbance in the heart's rhythm — usually require medication. Discuss the need for medication with your physician.

What Causes this Feeling of Fogginess I Have?

Several MVPers complain about this feeling. Some say they have a hard time remembering what they are supposed to remember, and feel as if they are in a daze. No one knows the reason. Some MVPers believe lack of sleep worsens their fogginess.

Can Smoking Make MVP Symptoms Worse?

Nicotine stimulates the sympathetic nervous system and affects the cardiovascular system. Theoretically, smoking can aggravate symptoms associated with MVPS. Also, cigarette smoking transiently increases the adhesiveness of platelets, accelerates the heart rate, and raises the blood-pressure. At the same time, the oxygen carrying capacity of the blood is reduced. Smoking is the leading cause of cardiovascular morbidity and mortality in the United States. It accounts for 30% to 40% of deaths from coronary artery disease. Smoking increases the incident of a heart attack and related death by 70%. For women taking oral contraceptives, cigarette smoking markedly predisposes to cardiovascular disease.

Smoking is the most preventable risk factor for cardiovascular disease.

Can I Live without Taking My Anti-anxiety Medication Such As Alprazolam (Xanax)?

Yes, of course you can.

No one has to take Xanax or other anti-anxiety medication. People who experience anxiety and panic attacks need to consciously and clearly establish priorities. If the highest priority in your life is not to take medication — especially none that is potentially addicting — then, aim to win the war against that evil and vile enemy ... Xanax. Use it only when you absolutely *have to*. Otherwise, you may feel defeated when you *do* use it, and become even more anxious about needing it again. This thought process increases your baseline anxiety level, and — in turn — increases the frequency of your panic attacks. To focus solely on the medication, you avoid the real causes of your anxiety and the games continue.

When you establish *yourself* as your top priority, and make *your* quality of life a goal, then Xanax, or other anti-anxiety medication, is useful as an aid. With your nervous system stabilized, and panic-attack symptoms controlled, you're better equipped — physically and emotionally — to consider the core issues that set your nervous system off like a brass band.

There are reasons for your panic attacks that you must address. First, however, the frightening and immobilizing symptoms have to be treated. Xanax, or similar medication, is effective short-term treatment for the symptoms. To rely on medication and to not address the cause of your symptoms is a disservice to you and the medication. Decide that YOU deserve something better in life.

References

Boudoulas, H., Kligfield, P. & Wooley, C. 1988. "Mitral valve prolapse: Sudden death." In: *Mitral Valve Prolapse and the Mitral Valve Prolapse Syndrome* (H. Boudoulas & C. Wooley, Eds.). Futura Publishing Co., Inc. Mount Kisco, NY. 591–605.

Dajani, A., Bisno, A., Chung, K. *et al.* 1990. "Prevention of bacterial endocarditis: Recommendations by the American Heart Association." *Journal of the American Medical Association.* **262:** (22), 2919–2922.

Devereux, R., Kramer-Fox, R., Shear, K., & Kligfield, P. 1994. "The relation of panic attacks and midsystolic murmurs to the diagnosis of mitral valve prolapse." *Cardiovascular Reviews & Reports.* **April:** 11–15, 34.

Eckman, J. (1991). Reader's Corner. *Network.* **3:** (1) 2.

Hussey, L. 1992. "What about Xanax? Part I." *Network.* **4:** (2) 1.

Kligfield, P., Levy, D., Devereux, R., *et al.* 1987. "Arrhythmias and sudden death in mitral valve prolapse." *American Heart Journal.* **113:** 1298–1307.

Kligfield, P. & Devereux, R. 1990. "Is the mitral valve prolapse patient at high risk of sudden death identifiable?" *Cardiovascular Clinics.* **21:** (1) 143–157.

Kolibash, A. 1988. "Natural history of mitral valve prolapse." In: *Mitral Valve Prolapse and the Mitral Valve Prolapse Syndrome* (Boudoulas, J, & Wooley, C., Eds.). Futura Publishing Co., Inc. Mount-Kisco, NY. 257–288.

Lax, D., Eicher, M. & Goldberg, S. 1993. "Effects of hydration on mitral valve prolapse." *American Heart Journal.* **126:** (2) 415–418.

Myerburg, R. & Castellanos, A. 1992. "Cardiac arrest and sudden cardiac death." In: *Heart Disease: A Textbook of Cardiovascular Medicine* (E. Braunwald, Ed.). 4th edit. 756–789. W.B. Saunders Co. Philadelphia.

Ohara, N., Mikajima, T., Takagi, J., & Kato, H. 1991. "Mitral valve prolapse in childhood: The incidence and clinical presentations in different age groups." *Acta Paediatri Jpn.* **336:** 467–475.

Savage, D., Garrison, R., Devereux, R., *et al.* (1983). Mitral valve prolapse in the general population. I. Epidemiologic features: The Framingham Study. *American Heart Journal.* **106:** 571–576.

Utz, S., & England, B. 1993. "Avoiding problems when taking antibiotics." *Network.* **5:** (3).

Summary

MVPS — mitral valve prolapse syndrome — a common clinical condition affects millions of people. Anatomic MVP — mitral valve prolapse — occurs when one or more mitral valve leaflets buckle back or prolapse into the left atrium as the heart contracts. Anatomic MVP is often associated with a constellation of symptoms, such as: fatigue, dizziness, palpitations, headaches, lightheadedness, chest pain, and panic attacks. Individuals with one or more of these symptoms are referred to as having mitral valve prolapse *syndrome*.

The term MVP syndrome refers to the occurrence of — or coexistence of — symptoms unexplainable on the basis of the valvular abnormality. *Thus, symptoms associated with MVPS are not due to the valve itself.* They are believed to be based on various physiological changes.

Often, these symptoms are frightening, discomforting, frustrating, and incapacitating. They can alter one's life-style, result in absenteeism from work, and cause disharmony within the family. Visits to an emergency room or a physician's office become quite common and nerve-racking.

Further research is needed to define methods of long-term treatment of MVPS. There are, however, non-drug interventions that effectively decrease the frequency and the severity of symptoms. Developed from information extrapolated from previous research studies, and from years of clinical experience, some recommendations include: regular cardiovascular exercise, an increase in sodium and fluid intake, and an avoidance of caffeine and over-the-counter medications that contain adrenaline-like substances.

In conclusion, this book provides you with information to better understand MVPS: what it is, what causes symptoms, and *what you can do to help yourself*. With knowledge comes power — the power to take control of your life. ***Now, Do It.***

About the Author

Dr. Kristine Scordo received her PhD and Master's degrees from The Ohio State University, undergraduate degrees from the University of Cincinnati and Mercy College, New York, and her RN diploma from Queens General Hospital, New York City. She is assistant professor, Wright State University–Miami Valley; clinical nurse specialist in cardiology; and clinical director of The Health Promotion and Rehabilitation Center and of The Mitral Valve Prolapse Program of Cincinnati. Dr. Scordo is a widely published author, editor, and lecturer.

Appendix:
Consumer Sources

For further information on various related health topics, contact one or more of the following organizations.

The Mitral Valve Prolapse Program of Cincinnati (MVPPC)
The Health Promotion and Rehabilitation Center
10525 Montgomery Road
Cincinnati, OH 45242
(513) 745-9911

MVPPC publishes a pamphlet on MVPS that gives a general overview of MVP, symptoms, antibiotic prophylaxis, and non-drug interventions. Single copies are available for free to consumers and health professionals. MVPPC also publishes a quarterly newsletter, *Network* ($20/year). The newsletter provides up-to-date information on MVPS, symptom-control measures, and answers questions from consumers. Back issues are available. Write or call for further information.

American Heart Association (AHA)
National Center 7320
Greenville Avenue Dallas, TX 75231
(214) 373-6300

The AHA provides a number of free pamphlets on a variety of health-related issues. These can be obtained from the National Center or from your local AHA chapter. Some of the publications-include:

American Heart Association Diet: Offers information about a fat-controlled, low cholesterol diet. One side of the pamphlet contains general information and the other side is a daily meal plan with recommendations of foods to avoid.

Recipes for Fat-Controlled, Low-Cholesterol Meals: This is the companion to the *AHA Diet* with sample recipes for satisfying and heart-healthy meals.

Nutritious Nibbles — Guide to Healthy Snacking: This publications discusses wise, nutritious, and enjoyable choices for snacking. Hints on certain foods to avoid, those to include, recipes, and tips for enjoying a calorie-free or low-calorie snack are given.

Nutrition Labeling — Food Selection Hints: Provides tips on how to read labels, guidelines for shopping for fat-controlled meals, and information about calories, cholesterol, and saturated fat.

Silent Epidemic: The Truth about Women and Heart Disease: This pamphlet, directed toward women, discusses heart disease, risk factors, methods of control, and steps toward prevention. It is intended to dispel the conception that heart disease is mainly a male problem.

Calling it Quits — Self-Help Smoking Cession Kit: This kit contains two booklets: *How to Quit*, an information booklet that provides a variety of tips on how to stop smoking; and *The Good Life* that suggests ways to cope with everyday urges to smoke.

"E" is for Exercise: Discusses the role of exercise in heart health, types of exercise, how to exercise, and factors to consider before undertaking an exercise program.

Nutrition for the Fitness Challenge: This publication addresses the nutritional requirements of a physically active individual. Information about protein, carbohydrates, fat, vitamins, minerals, and water is given. Contains a food guide for physical fitness and cardiovascular health.

Safeguarding Your Heart During Pregnancy: This pamphlet is written for women with a history of heart disease, valve replacement, heart murmur, or rheumatic fever who is pregnant or considering pregnancy. It discusses normal changes in the circulatory system during pregnancy, effects of heart disease on childbearing, cardiac ailments acquired during pregnancy, and drug therapy.

Cycling for a Healthy Heart, Dancing for a Healthy Heart, Running for a Healthy Heart, Swimming for a Healthy Heart, and Walking for a Healthy Heart: All are brochures that provide information about the benefits of exercise, how to begin a specific exercise program, and how to monitor progress.

American Dietetic Association (ADA)
430 North Michigan Avenue
Chicago, IL 60611
(312) 280-5000

The ADA offers cookbooks and other materials which are designed to educate the consumer about food and nutrition.

The Dieter's Guide ($4.00) and *Eating the Moderate Fat and Cholesterol Way* ($2.50) provide information on low-calorie recipes.

Audiocassettes on topics such as coping with job-related stress are also available.

American Psychiatric Association
1400 K Street, N.W.
Washington, D.C. 20005
(202) 682-6000

Pamphlets that discuss the recognition and treatment of various mental-health issues such as anxiety, depression, and phobias are available by contacting the APA Division of Public Affairs. Single copies of the pamphlets are available for free.

American Self-Help Clearinghouse
Saint Clares-Riverside Medical Center
25 Pocono Road
Denville, New Jersey 07834
(210) 625-7101

American Self-Help Clearinghouse publishes *Sourcebook*, a national guide to finding and forming mutual aid self-help groups. The book contains over 700 national and model self-help groups that cover a broad range of addictions, disabilities, illnesses, patenting concerns, bereavement, and many other stressful life situation.

Cerenex™ Pharmaceuticals
Division of Glaxo, Inc.
Five Moore Drive
Research Triangle Park
North Carolina 27709

Cerenex publishes a quarterly newsletter designed to provide migraine sufferers with up-to-date information about migraine. Issues highlight tips for living with migraine and new research.

Obtain a free subscription by writing to: Headway, PO Box 9147, Opalocka, FL 33054-9893.

Consumer Information Center
Pueblo, CO 81009

The *Consumer Information Catalog* lists over 200 booklets on consumer topics including high blood pressure, sodium, fats and cholesterol, and weight control. Write for a free copy.

Food and Drug Administration (FDA)
Office of Consumer Affairs, HFE-88
5600 Fishers Lane
Rockville, MD 20857
(301) 443-3170

The FDA offers a variety of publications on topics such as general drug information and food-related subjects including cholesterol. The FDA publishes a monthly journal, *FDA Consumer* that reports on various health issues. Contact the above address to obtain the phone number of the consumer affairs office nearest you. Single copies of publications are free.

National Heart, Lung, and Blood Institute (NHLBI)
Office of Prevention, Education, and Control
Communications and Public Information Branch
Building 31, Room 4A21
Bethesda, MD 20892
(301) 496-4236

The NHLBI offers a variety of free consumer publications, a nutrition fact book called *Eaters' Almanac*, and a quiz entitled *Test Your Healthy Heart I*. The NHLBI also offers a number of fact sheets including:

Facts about ... Women, Heart Disease, and Stroke: This publication offers information on the three major risk factors for heart disease — elevated blood cholesterol, high blood pressure, and cigarette smoking. Data on prevalence, risk, and treatment benefits are included.

Facts about ... Exercise: What is Fact and What is Fiction?: This publication discusses common myths about exercise and explains how regular physical activity can reduce some risk factors for heart disease.

Facts about … Exercise: Sample Exercise Programs: This discusses how to avoid exercise-related injuries and includes sample walking and jogging programs.

Facts about … Blood Cholesterol: This publication discusses blood cholesterol, its importance as a risk factor for coronary heart disease, the benefits of reducing blood cholesterol,-and the role of saturated fat and dietary cholesterol.

National Headache Foundation
5252 North Western Avenue
Chicago, Illinois 60625
(312) 878-5558 or (800) 843-2256

Offers information on headaches: causes and treatment. For the publication, *The Headache Handbook*, include a business-size, self-addressed, stamped envelope with $.50.

National Health Information Clearinghouse (NHIC)
1255 23rd Street, NW
Suite 275
Washington, DC 20037
(800) 336-4797 or
(202) 429-9091 in the Washington metropolitan area

The NHIC is a central source of information and referral for health-related questions of consumers and health professionals. Questions are answered with publications directly from its library or by referral to appropriate agencies. The NHIC develops and distributes *Healthfinders* ($1.00), a periodical publication on selected health topics. Publications' lists are available.

National Institute of Mental Health
5600 Fishers Lane
Rockville, MD 20857
(301) 443-4536

Call 1-800-64-PANIC for free publications on panic disorder, its diagnosis, treatment, and for referrals.

National Mental Health Association (NMHA)
61021 Price Street
Alexandria, Virginia 22314-2971
(703) 684-7722

The NMHA offers a variety of publications that address mental health. Some of these include Stress: *A Fact of Life, Coping: Get-*

ting Help When You Need It, and *A Teenager's Guide to Surviving Stress*. These pamphlets discuss what stress is, helpful hints on managing stress, and where people can seek further assistance. Write or call for a list of their publications.

Office on Smoking and Health (OSH)
Park Building
Room 110 (for publications)
Room 116 (for Technical Information Center)
5600 Fishers Lane
Rockville, MD 20857
(301) 443-1575

The OSH serves as a clearing-house on information about smoking. Pamphlets include *Pregnant? That's Two Good Reasons to Quit Smoking*, and discusses benefits of not smoking during pregnancy and breast feeding. Health statistics and reports such as *The Health Consequences of Smoking for Women* are also available. Materials are free.

White Light Yoga
Sara Harris
4 City Hall Road
Accord, New York 12404
(914) 626-2843

Sara Harris has given experiential lectures to corporate groups and organizations on *Inner Developmental* techniques since 1972. She is a stress management lecturer and a certified yoga therapist, providing professional programs year round. Sara has produced reputable meditation tapes and an excellent video for beginner and intermediate yoga practitioners. More information and an order form can be obtained by calling (leave a message with your name and address) or by writing to Sara Harris.

Questionnaire ■

As an MVPer, your input is important to help us learn more about this syndrome. Please take a few minutes to complete the following questionnaire.

1. At what age were you diagnosed with MVPS ?

_____ not diagnosed   _____ 18 or under   _____ 19 to 25   _____ 26 to 35

_____ 36 to 45   _____ 46 to 55   _____ 56 to 65   _____ 66 or older

2. Please check any symptoms that first caused you to consult with a physician.

_____ chest pain   _____ palpitations   _____ tachycardia

_____ skipped heartbeat   _____ extra beats   _____ dizziness

_____ passing out   _____ headaches   _____ fatigue

_____ lightheadedness   _____ panic attacks   _____ anxiety

_____ mood swings   _____ shortness of breath   _____ other: _____

3. At what age did you first begin to experience these symptoms?

_____ 18 or under   _____ 19 to 25   _____ 26 to 35   _____ 36 to 45

_____ 46 to 55   _____ 56 to 65   _____ 66 or older

4. Prior to your diagnosis of MVP, were you ever diagnosed with another medical condition that was later ruled out?   _____ yes   _____ no
If yes, what was the diagnosis?   _____

5. Please place a check to indicate you have the following:

_____ click   _____ murmur   _____ echocardiogram showing MVP

6. Please check any symptoms you once had, plus any you have.

_____ chest pain   _____ palpitations   _____ tachycardia

_____ skipped heartbeat   _____ extra beats   _____ dizziness

_____ passing out   _____ shortness of breath   _____ problems sleeping

_____ headaches   _____ fatigue   _____ lightheadedness

_____ panic attacks   _____ anxiety   _____ mood swings

_____ arm pain   _____ cold hands/feet   _____ stomach problems

_____ other: _____

7. Please list your current medications: _____

_____

8. What worsens your symptoms?

_____ alcohol   _____ emotional stress   _____ foods: specify _____

_____ over exertion   _____ menses   _____

_____ lack of sleep   _____ being fatigued   _____ other:_____

_____ caffeine

9. What lessens your symptoms?

_____ avoiding caffeine   _____ avoiding stress   _____ balanced diet

_____ regular exercise   _____ increased water intake   _____ adequate rest

_____ other: _____

10. Were your symptoms preceded by a major stressor? _____ yes _____ no
If yes, was it:

_____ marriage   _____ divorce   _____ death of a family member

_____ menopause   _____ personal illness   _____ job change

_____ other: _____

11. Within the past year, please indicate the number of times your symptoms:

_____ caused you to visit the emergency room

_____ caused you to visit your physician

Please let us know what you think about *Taking Control*.
1. What feature did you like the most?
_____

2. What feature could be omitted?
_____

3. What questions, issues, or topics would you like to have discussed in future editions?_____

How did you find out about this book? _____

What is your age?

_____ 18 or under   _____ 19 to 25   _____ 26 to 35   _____ 36 to 45

_____ 46 to 55   _____ 56 to 65   _____ 66 or older

What is your sex ? _____ male   _____ female

To receive a complimentary copy of *Network*, the newsletter from The MVP Program of Cincinnati, please provide us with your name and address.

Name: _____

Address: _____

City: _____State: _____ Zip Code: _____

Thank you for helping other MVPers by responding to this survey. Please return your completed questionnaire to:

MVP Questionnaire
c/o K.A. Scordo
P.O. Box 626
Loveland, OH 45140

Subject Index

A

acetylcholine, 13
adrenalin (see also epinephrine, catecholamines), 13, 53, 60
aerobic dance
    high impact, 84
    low impact, 84
    shoes, 85
aerobic exercise, 72, 75
    effects of, long term, 73
    effects of, short term, 72
    exammples, 72
    signs of improvement (list), 96
air bike, 85
alcohol, 5, 12, 16, 29, 169
aldosterone, 14–15
alpha receptor, 150
Alprazolam (Xanax), 173
American Dietetic Association (ADA), 179
American Heart Association, 159, 177
American Psychiatric Association, 179
American Self-Help Clearinghouse, 179
amoxicillin, 160
anaerobic exercise, 73
anatomic mitral valve prolapse, 2
    primary, 4
angina, 4
angiogram, 32
antacids, 161
antiarrhythmic drugs, 153
antibiotic prophylaxis, 59, 162, 166
    use in children, 160
antibiotics, 158, 159, 160, 172
    helpful hints when taking (list), 161
antidepressants, 122
antihistamines, 168
anxiety (see also panic attacks), 113–115, 117–119, 121, 169, 173
    anticipatory, 110
    baseline level, 127
    chronic, 117
    definition of, 109
    frequently asked questions about, 123–128

anxiety —continued
    reduction with carbohydrates, 126
anxiety agents, anti-, 120,123
anxiety attack, 108, 110
    and caffiene, 48
    at night, 125
anxiety disorder, 17
arm ergometer, 86
arm, back, or shoulder discomfort, 11
arm span, 2
arrhythmias, 5, 7, 8
    cardiac, 16
    detecting, 7
    types of, 9
Ativan (lorezepam), 26, 37, 123
atria, 6, 7, 9
atrial beat (contraction), premature, 7
atrial fibrillation (see also arrhythmmias), 9
autonomic nervous system (see also sympathetic nervous system), 13, 14, 21
    dysfunction, 13
autonomic testing, 19–20

B

bargaining, 44, 45, 46
Barlow's Syndrome, 2
beta blockers (see also medications), 17, 23, 43, 149, 150, 152, 154, 155
    and exercise, 155
    in combination with channel blockers, 153
    interaction with other medications, 152
    list of, 151
    possible side effects of, 152
    predictable effects of, 151
beta receptors, 150
bicycle ergometers, 87
bicycling outside, 87
bioavailability, 59
birth control pills, risks of, 165
Blockadren (timolol), 151
blood pressure, 15, 18, 20
blood, donating, 165
blurred vision, 10